Body Conditioning, Figure and Weight Control for Women

Maryhelen Vannier

Southern Methodist University

Wadsworth Publishing Company, Inc.
Belmont, California

CONTENTS

1 VALUES — 1

2 HISTORY — 3

3 HOW FIT ARE YOU REALLY? — 5

4 FIND YOUR BODY TYPE AND SET YOUR FIGURE IMPROVEMENT GOALS — 14

5 NUTRITION AND TOTAL FITNESS — 21

6 SLIMNASTIC EXERCISES — 31

Body Conditioning Exercises — 32
Exercises for the Waistline — 34
Exercises for the Hips and Thighs — 40
Exercises for the Bust, Chest, and Arms — 45
Exercises for the Feet and Ankles — 48
Exercises for Posture Improvement — 50
Yoga Relaxation Exercises — 52
Exercises to Relieve Menstrual Pain — 56
Exercises for the Neck, Face, and Chin — 59
Exercises to Make You Feel Good — 60

7 HOW TO STAY SLIM AND TRIM FOR LIFE — 62

8 GLOSSARY — 65

9 BIBLIOGRAPHY — 67

L. C. Cat. Card No. 72-91612   Printed in the United States of America.

ISBN-0-534-00133-5

1 2 3 4 5 6 7 8 9 10—77 76 75 74 73

VALUES

Our push-button society with its modern work saving devices is robbing people of physical activity. American women want desperately to have sleek, trim, attractive figures, but few of them know how to accomplish it — they seek a quick, easy way to become shapely: expensive reducing salons, slenderizing belts, exercise machines, and other widely advertised gadgets, which produce negligible permanent results. Popular crash diets leave women malnourished, irritable, and disillusioned. One of the best ways to build and maintain body efficiency and physical fitness is to engage in a vigorous, daily body exercise program that is fun, challenging, and rewarding. Although exercise is not a panacea, when it is coupled with good nutrition and healthful recreation it can transform a wilted daisy into a tiger lily.

Your body needs activity just as it needs food. Inactivity adds weight and drains energy; exercise will help you to become attractive and vigorous. Don't fear that increased activity will make you eat more and gain weight — according to medical experts just the opposite is true. As you take part in a structured exercise program you will discover that a glass of water can allay your hunger pangs. Exercise can relieve your tensions and smooth unattractive bulges and sags. You will succeed only by giving up your old habits, applying yourself to a new regime, and realizing that if you don't look after your body, no one else will.

Many women fear that with weight loss they will have slack breasts, and sagging upper arms, thighs, and hips. Again, the opposite is true. The body will be firmer and more shapely, provided that you do specific exercises to build muscle firmness. When you lose weight, you are shedding the water between body tissues and the fat from the fatty layers just under the skin; consequently you must actively engage in specific exercises for those body areas. You should follow the exercises in this booklet for trimming hips and thighs, waist and back, legs and ankles, arms and shoulders, neck and chin. In addition you can do rhythmical, relaxing exercises to reduce your tensions and lift your spirits.

The most assured way to have an attractive body is to eat less and exercise more. Two experts, a physiologist and a physical educator, point out:

The use of physical activity to promote weight loss in overweight people has been dismissed by some professional people because they feel that the amount of exercise required to metabolize fat tissue is far in excess of that which is practical in any reasonable exercise program. One pound of fat has an equivalency of over 4,000 kilocalories, and on this basis, in order to lose a pound of fat, one must play tennis for 9 hours, play volleyball for 11 hours or walk for 21 hours. However, such logic is faulty because it is not only unnecessary but physiologically undesirable to lose weight in a short period of time. Most *physicians recommend the loss of only one or two pounds per week as a rule of thumb,* and this is entirely compatible within the levels of energy expenditure involved in physical activity. With a suitable exercise program it is possible to burn off only fractions of that pound of fat during each exercise session. These fractions can gradually accumulate over a period of months and, if caloric intake is held relatively constant, a sizeable weight loss can be incurred.[1]

[1]Fred Roby and Russell Davis, *Jogging for Fitness and Weight Control* (Philadelphia: W. B. Saunders, 1970), p. 23.

HISTORY 2

Eve knew how to attract Adam; Greek goddesses are legendary beauties; Grecian and Roman art show us beautifully proportioned statues of women, and the rich tapestries of the Middle Ages portray in multicolored threads the lovely, fragile, noble ladies of that period. American women historically were powerful pioneers — both childbearers and supporters of the nation's morale. Only after the country was won, the family raised and gone, and the food larder full, did Americans begin to think of the "good life" as softer, less exerting. Now history's pendulum is swinging away from the concept of the "soft life" to a more vigorous, productive life. Modern women are not content to be beautiful, fragile butterflies, displayed for men to admire, protected from life. Today American women want to become *involved* in life. In ever increasing numbers they are "doers" rather than "watchers" of life. Women's liberation movements have succeeded in alerting women to the active and productive role they might play in improving their existences.

In 1941, Americans were shocked to learn that many young men inducted into military service were rejected for health reasons or physical handicaps. People gradually became aware that the young as well as the middle-aged were not as sound physically as they should be. In the early 1950s research conducted in the U.S. and Europe showed that well fed, inactive American children were inferior in physical strength and body endurance and flexibility levels to more active European youth. As a result, in 1956 President Eisenhower formed the Physical Fitness Commission to increase interest and effort for building a vigorous, national youth fitness program.

President Kennedy gave the greatest impetus to physical fitness programs for people of all ages. Today more people than ever before are jogging, playing golf, bowling, bicycling, and playing other kinds of vigorous sports and games. Leading medical authorities such as Dr. Paul Dudley White, the famous heart specialist, have done much to convince Americans that inactivity and heart disease are linked. We have discovered the health-giving value of play and know that we can become stronger, more vigorous, and healthier by an increased participation in sports and a program of daily physical exercise.

Physical education today is increasingly regarded as a vital part of general education. The ancient Greeks recognized physical activity as an aid to medicine and health. Hippocrates, the ancient Greek physician, stressed the law of "use," claiming that through use (exercise), all parts of the body become strong and healthy, whereas disuse (lack of exercise) results in imperfect development, body deterioration, and illness. Plato believed that a good education consisted of permitting the body and the soul to achieve all the beauty and perfection of which they are capable. Aristotle held that the body and soul were interrelated, as mental and physical health are closely allied. Have a "sound mind in a sound body" declared John Locke, the famous English philosopher. And the Bible frequently counsels that the body should be cared for since it houses the soul.

Just as primitive man had to learn to use his body wisely or perish, so must we. In our tension filled, overpopulated, fast moving society, we may need vigorous physical activity more than ever before. Work balanced with exercise and recreation improves health and happiness. The human body will serve its owner well only if it is kept in good working order. Unfortunately too many overfed, underexercised Americans take better care of their cars than they do of their bodies.

HOW FIT ARE YOU REALLY? 3

We change throughout our lives. Daily changes affect how you look and feel, act, think, work, and play.

Your body is like a machine — it must be kept in the best possible working order. Your present health affects your future fitness. Good health should be carefully sought after and maintained. Fitness is the product of habit and a determined desire to keep it. Learning how to relax and to keep your body in the best condition will take persistence and *consistent* effort *every* day.

Your body is composed of 639 muscles and 208 bones, millions of tissues, and hundreds of moving parts. It can only increase its strength, efficiency, and beauty with vigorous activity and a well-balanced, controlled diet. To *gain* increased physical energy, you must *spend* increased physical effort.

WHAT IS PHYSICAL FITNESS?

Total fitness (emotional, spiritual, physical, and nutritional) cannot be stored for future use, but must be continually replenished. Vigorous physical activity — more than that required for work and the daily simple life movements — is necessary to develop an attractive, efficient body. Healthy, zestful individuals are also highly motivated, vital people. Unless you remain active, walk more and drive less, eat properly, and have creative leisure time outlets, your firmness will become flabby with age. Fitness is individual; it enables your body to function at a high level of efficiency. The eminent physiologist, Arthur Steinhaus, has defined fitness as:

1. A body free from disease.

2. Muscles, heart, and lungs developed to give strength.

3. An alert mind, free from undue worry, that can relax with the moment of opportunity and as quickly be engrossed in the next challenging task.

4. A spirit that feels itself unselfishly part of an important venture and important to that venture.[2]

I would include these other two qualities of fitness:

5. You do not deviate markedly from normal body weight in relationship to your age, height, and body frame (small, average, or heavy).

6. You have enough strength and endurance to do your daily work without excessive fatigue and still have an emergency strength reserve.

The American Medical Association contends that the seven paths to fitness are good medical care, regular dental care, proper eating habits, exercise, enjoyable work, healthful play, and rest and relaxation.[3] You and your physician can determine if you are as fit as you should be, have enough strength and stamina, and take part in sufficient daily physical activity to live productively and happily in our highly competitive, work oriented society.

If you have ever been confined to bed for a few days, you know how quickly strength diminishes. Just as unused silver tarnishes quickly, your body becomes ugly, weak and flabby when not used properly. The longer you stay inactive, the longer it will take to trim and reshape you figure.

Can you pinch more than an inch of flesh around your upper arms, waist, hips, or sides? Stand nude before a long mirror. Do you sag? Where? How much? Take a deep breath, pull in your stomach, tighten all your muscles. Do you feel the difference between body flabbiness and firmness?

Answer the following questions:

Yes No

— — 1. Do you usually wake up in the morning feeling tired and achy?

— — 2. Do you generally have a hard time going to sleep at night?

— — 3. Are you "potty," "hippy," "saggy"?

— — 4. Are you often jittery, nervous, weepy?

— — 5. Are you often worried, moody? Are your moods extreme?

[2] Arthur Steinhaus, *How to Keep Fit and Like It* (Chicago: The Dartnell Corporation, 1957).

[3] American Medical Association, *Seven Paths to Fitness* (Chicago: American Medical Association, 1967).

—— —— 6. Can you relax when you feel tension rising in the back of you neck and shoulders?
—— —— 7. Do you have frequent headaches?
—— —— 8. Are you often constipated? Do you often have bad breath or frequent indigestion after eating?
—— —— 9. Do you have frequent colds, joint pains, aching feet?
—— —— 10. Does climbing a flight of stairs leave you breathless?
—— —— 11. Do people frequently "bug" you?
—— —— 12. Do you eat three well-balanced meals every day?
—— —— 13. Do you often snack between meals?
—— —— 14. Do you take tranquilizers, pep pills, stimulants, or sleeping pills?

If you answered "no" to all items except 6 and 12, you take good care of your body and have good health habits. If you answered "yes" to any other questions, you need to begin *now* to change your habits and improve your health.

QUICK AND REVEALING FITNESS TESTS

Another quick way to discover how fit you really are is to run or swim vigorously for as long as you can. If you are in good physical condition, you should be able to alternate a run-walk for at least 12 minutes without being utterly exhausted, or swim for 8 minutes continuously without stopping to rest.

Other quick tests of your present physical fitness:

	Poor	*Average*	*Good*	*Superior*
1. *Balance.* Standing on one foot with your eyes open, and hands out for balance, rise to your toes holding free leg forward. Do not shift your weighted foot.	14 seconds	20 seconds	44 seconds	60 seconds
2. *Flexibility.* Stand with your feet 12 inches apart. Keep your knees straight, bend forward and touch the floor.	Cannot touch the floor	Can barely touch with fingertips	Can touch the floor with fingertips with ease	Can touch your palms to the floor
3. *Flexibility.* Lying face down on the floor with	12 inches	18 inches	22 inches	26 inches

your fingers laced behind your neck (with or without someone holding your feet), raise your upper body as far off the floor as you can.

	Cannot touch fingers	Can touch fingers	Can lock fingers	Can fully grasp fingers, hands
4. *Flexibility.* Reach your right hand over your right shoulder with your palm in; reach your left hand around back with palm out. Grasp hands behind your back.	Cannot touch fingers	Can touch fingers	Can lock fingers	Can fully grasp fingers, hands
5. *Strength.* Stand with your feet apart and do stride jumps (alternate feet together then apart for count 1) for 25 up and back, then up and down in place. Repeat.	150 times	300 times	450 times	600 times
6. *Strength.* Lying face down with your palms on the floor under your shoulders, push up until arms and body are straight. Repeat.	Less than 8 times	8 times	14 times	20 times
7. *Endurance.* Run in place for 60 seconds at 180 steps per minute. Take a deep breath and hold it as long as you can.	10 seconds	20 seconds	30 seconds	45 seconds
8. *Endurance.* Run around a basketball court at a moderately fast pace.	5 times	10 times	15 times	20 times
9. *Endurance and strength.* Lying flat on your back with knees bent and fingers laced behind your neck, rise to a straight sitting position. Have a partner hold your feet down, if necessary.	10 times	20 times	35 times	50 times

OTHER QUICK AND REVEALING FITNESS TESTS[4]

1. On the balls of your feet, jump from behind a line by bending your

[4] These items test balance, flexibility, agility, strength, power, and endurance. They have been selected from T. Cureton's "A Stiff But Reliable Test of Fitness," *The Healthy Life* (New York: Time-Life Books, 1966), p. 18.

knees and swinging both arms back, then forward to give you power. Record your best distance of 3 tries. You should jump at least 6 feet 7 inches.

2. Spread your hands the width of your shoulders, and curl your fingers toward you around a chinning bar or tree limb; pull your body up from full extension until your chin is over the bar. Keep your body straight. If you have good physical strength, you can hang 55 seconds or longer.

3. With your shoulders back and your chest expanded, measure the circumference of your chest just below your armpits. Then measure your waist with your stomach in a relaxed position. Your chest should measure 5 inches more than your waist.

4. Sit on the floor with your legs stretched out in front of you, and place a book 8 inches tall upright between your knees. Then, keeping your legs straight and flat on the floor, bend forward from the waist and touch your forehead to the top of the book. Do this once to see how flexible you are.

5. Stand on your toes with your heels together, your eyes closed, and your arms fully extended. Stay in this position for 20 seconds without shifting your feet or opening your eyes.

6. Lie on your back with your hands clasped behind your neck, and raise both legs to a vertical position without bending them. Repeat this 20 times successively.

7. With your body stretched sideways, support yourself on one hand (with your arm held straight) and the outside of one foot. Place your other hand on your hip. Raise your upper leg to a horizontal position 25 times without bending either knee.

8. Run in place for 60 seconds, lifting your feet at least 4 inches from the floor. Take 3 deep breaths; then hold your breath for 30 seconds.

If you can perform all these tests you are probably in as good physical condition as you should be.

EFFECTS OF PHYSICAL ACTIVITY

If you have discovered from these tests that you are not as physically fit as you should be, set up a vigorous physical exercise program of 30 minutes *daily* and *stick to it*. If you are overweight or if your body is flabby do something about it.

The key factors in any exercise program are *duration* (exercise long enough to produce increased circulation until you are perspiring and gasping for breath), *intensity* (begin gradually, increase speed, then taper off), and *frequency* (exercise briskly 30 minutes daily after you attain good condition). The following facts about exercise and the benefit of daily vigorous physical activity will help you understand the value of the exercise program.

Exercise

1. Helps keep weight normal when coupled with reduced food intake and no between meal snacks.

2. Increases muscular strength, physical endurance, and attractiveness.

3. Improves circulation and produces more red blood corpuscles so that all body cells are given the best kind of nourishment.

4. Increases heart strength, thus reducing the chances of heart attack.

5. Relieves tension and fatigue by providing an outlet for feelings of hostility and aggression, thus helping to prevent psychosomatic illness.

6. Increases the function of all body systems, especially those of circulation, respiration, and digestion. You feel healthy.

7. Increases neuromuscular coordination. Movements become more skillful and productive.

8. Produces greater strength and resiliency of the skeletal system by increasing the size and thickness of bones.

9. Builds resistance to disease and fatigue.

10. Stimulates physical growth and redistributes weight and body fat.

11. Favorably affects the cooperative tasks of the internal body organs and glands and increases the efficiency for the assigned tasks of each one.

12. Helps remove more quickly body waste products through perspiration, respiration, and elimination.

13. Provides a youthful and zestful feeling throughout life by retarding both physical and mental effects of aging.

14. Increases the recovery rate after surgery and major illness.

15. Aids in easing childbirth and in regaining an attractive figure after childbirth.

16. Helps make sleep more refreshing.

17. Prevents the weakening of the abdominal wall, thus preventing a "pot belly."

18. Leads to quick recovery from fatigue following strenuous activity; helps in developing the ability to do more on less breath, which is especially advantageous to an athlete.

CARDIOVASCULAR BENEFITS OF EXERCISE

Through vigorous exercise your lungs process more air with less effort, your heart becomes stronger, pumps more blood with fewer strokes, and increases your total blood volume, according to Kenneth Cooper. Blood pressure and recovery rate following strenuous exercise are also influenced by regular physical activity. Dr. Cooper has developed a famous scientific physical fitness program called Aerobics which is based upon a point system. The participant in this program keeps track of points on a weekly basis for running, swimming, cycling, walking, stationary running, and for playing handball, squash, or basketball. The program depends on the individual's physical fitness category based on the distance run in 12 minutes according to the following scale:[5]

The 12-Minute Run

If you cover	You are in this fitness category
less than 1.0 mile	I Very poor
1.0 to 1.24 miles	II Poor
1.25 to 1.49 miles	III Fair
1.50 to 1.74 miles	IV Good
1.75 miles or more	V Excellent

Principle of Overload and Adaptation.   The muscles become stronger and more efficient in their intended work when they are exercised progressively harder. Exercise periods should gradually be increased in speed and duration to produce "overload" of the muscles, thus augmenting their stamina and strength.

BECOME FIT AND ENJOY LIFE MORE

Good health is essential for success in all phases of life. Follow a vigorous·

---

[5] Kenneth Cooper, *Aerobics* (New York: Bantam Books, 1968), p. 1.

daily exercise routine, couple it with a controlled diet of three well-balanced meals every day; use brisker movements in your daily tasks and you will become revitalized, happier, and more productive — you can do more in less time and do it better. The following suggestions will help you reach a greater degree of total fitness:

1. Walk more, ride less. Climb steps, rather than riding the elevator. Use your legs! Pump more blood through your body and give strength to your heart muscle. Blow out the cobwebs by picking up speed as you move.

2. Pull in your stomach, tighten your buttocks, and hold yourself in as long as you can. Do this exercise often during the day (when you comb your hair, brush your teeth, talk over the phone).

3. S-T-R-E-T-C-H and try to touch the top of the door jamb in any room. Tighten your entire body and keep it taut while you slowly count to ten as you are in this stretched, taut position.

EXERCISE DOS AND DON'TS

Remember that the proper kind and amount of exercise (which affects shape) must be accompanied by a well-controlled diet (which affects weight).

Do: set aside 20 minutes each day for exercising at first. Make your exercise program as habitual as brushing your teeth.

Do: exercise to music with a strong 4/4 beat and a sprightly tune. (See Bibliography for list of recordings of directions for exercising.) Music makes exercising more fun.

Do: begin gradually, doing 8 to 10 minutes for the first several days; then increasing your time to 20 minutes or more as soon as you can. If you can do 20 minutes with ease, gradually increase this amount to a longer time.

Do: wear shorts or slacks, and loose fitting undergarments. Whenever possible, exercise barefooted.

Do: start with warm-up exercises; then do exercises to increase strength and flexibility; finally do the endurance exercises.

Do: if possible, shower briskly and rub down after exercise.

Do: couple your daily exercise program with brisk walking and other outdoor activities. Breathe deeply as you move about.

Don't: begin an exercise program until you have had a complete physical examination, or at least a heart checkup.

Don't: expect magical results overnight. Your body has been in its present condition for years; it cannot be refashioned in a few days or weeks.

Don't: try to push yourself too far or too fast.

Don't: skip days. Exercise vigorously for 20 minutes or more *every* day. Exercise must become a habit.

FIND YOUR BODY TYPE AND SET YOUR FIGURE IMPROVEMENT GOALS 4

Three of every ten Americans are from 10 to 20 pounds overweight. Serious obesity affects 25 percent of all Americans. Obesity is a vicious circle: the fatter you are the more you eat; the more you eat, the fatter you get; the fatter you are the shorter your life expectancy. The cycle begins with stress, anxiety, and tension resulting in compulsive eating; overeating leads to obesity, then to inactivity, and soon reverts to emotional stress. Obesity places a heavy burden on the entire body — the feet and legs, the internal organs, and especially on the heart. Experiment by carrying a 10 pound bag of sugar (as if you were 10 pounds overweight) for 30 minutes. See how tired you get? Imagine, then, carrying this extra load every day and estimate what that would do to you over a period of time.

Heart disease, the chief cause of death in America, is mostly due to obesity, increased stress, and insufficient exercise.[6] If you control your diet and weight, learn how to avoid, as well as to cope with tension, and follow a vigorous 30-minute daily exercise program designed for you, you may live longer and enjoy life more.

It is simple to have an attractive figure and good health. Let me repeat: the *only* scientific approach to weight reduction and figure reshaping lies in a program of diet control and increased exercise. Again, crash diets — be they milk, grapefruit, banana, Mayo, or any other current fad — will bring only temporary water loss and often permanent and dangerous results.

The units of fuel in food are called calories. To do our daily work well we each need an amount appropriate for us, depending on the kind of work we do, and our body type. We become too thin if we eat too little and overweight if we eat more than we burn up. A moderately active adult of normal weight burns between 14 to 20 calories a day for each pound of body weight. The more active you are, the more calories you burn.

We eat because we need food. But we also eat to be sociable or to

---

[6]William Raab, "Heart Attack—Number One Killer of Americans," *The Healthy Life* (New York: Time-Life Books, 1966), pp. 18-25.

distract ourselves from our troubles. Overeating and underexercising are the chief causes of obesity. The former is due largely to psychological needs (about 95 per cent), and rarely to physiological needs (only about 5 per cent). Overstuffing the body may be due to long-standing family habits. If you come from a family of "big eaters," notice how many of them become big people, and bigger yearly, as they keep eating as much (when they need less energy and food) as they did when they were younger, still growing, and more active. If you want to be thin, refuse to join the "oral gratifiers" who gorge themselves on food. Like alcoholism, obesity is linked with emotional problems that quickly become physical ones.

Like alcoholics, overweight overeaters:

Resent people's telling them that they eat or drink too much.

Try to get more food and drink than other guests at parties.

Indulge themselves between meals with frequent snacks.

Have a snack or drink before parties where they know food and drink will be served.

Envy those who can eat or drink more than they can without gaining weight.

Blame overindulgence on overactive thyroid glands or abnormal body requirements.

Insist that they can diet whenever they really want to.

FIND YOUR BODY TYPE

Does your body most resemble: a square, a pencil, or an inverted triangle? Pinch yourself around the middle, hips, upper arms, and sides. If your flesh feels firm, you have good muscle tone. If it is flabby, you have work to do. If you fear that exercise will make you appear muscular, remember that behind every curve there must be a well-proportioned muscle.

Every woman has her own body build (*somatotype*), depending on her muscularity, linearity, and fat distribution.

The three main body types are:

The Endomorph (the big square): This type is square-shaped, has a large frame, and is well padded with fat around the stomach, hips, upper arms, and neck. She usually has small hands and feet, short arms and legs. Because of her excessive bulk, she moves slowly, has slow reaction time, and tends to be sluggish. Her weight will be a problem throughout her life.

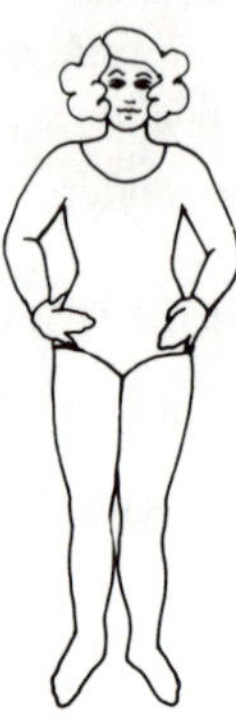

The Mesomorph (inverted triangle): This type has a firm, well proportioned body with broader shoulders than hips. She is usually active, likes sports, and tends to excel in those which require balance, endurance, strength, and speed.

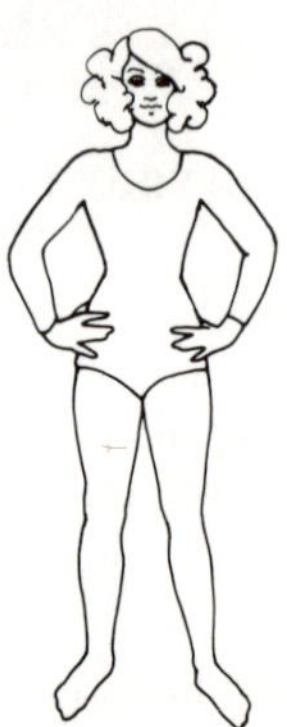

The Ectomorph (frail, pencil-thin): This type has a long, thin body with underdeveloped muscles, sloping shoulders, a low waistline, long arms and legs. Less strenuous individual sports appeal to her more than more active team games. She tires easily and may eat well, but will likely remain thin and wiry throughout her life.

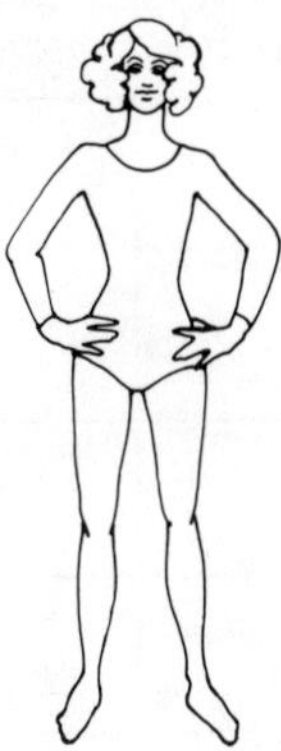

Although your body frame is inherited and unchanging, you can control the amount of flesh on that frame, and how attractive you will be by how much you eat and how much physical activity you regularly engage in.

The size of the internal organs is in direct proportion to each unique body. According to Eldon Shelton, an eminent authority on Somatotyping, each body type also has its own temperament and particular personality.

FIND YOUR BODY MEASUREMENTS

The well-proportioned body:

1. Waistline is 8-10 inches smaller than bust (measured at fullest part).

2. Slim hips should measure the same as the bust, full hips measure 3-4 inches larger (hips measured at largest part of buttocks).

3. Calf (measured at largest part of the lower leg) is 4-5 inches larger than ankle.

4. Ankles are 10-13 inches smaller than thighs.[7]

[7] Janet Wessel, *Movement Fundamentals, Figure, Form, Fun* (Englewood Cliffs, N.J.: Prentice-Hall, Inc., 1971), p. 39.

Using a measuring tape, measure your neck, upper arms, waist, thighs, and ankles. Record your measurements on a chart like the one below. In the right column write the measurements you want to achieve. Record your weight reduction weekly and your weight distribution monthly.

	Present Measurement	1st Month	2nd Month	3rd Month	4th Month	Goal
Neck: Just under chin	12¼"					
Bust: At fullest part	32"					
Waist: At narrowest part	24½					
Arm: Close to armpit	9¾					
Thigh: At largest part	21¾					
Calf: At largest part	14½					

Next, check your height and weight according to the following charts:

Desirable Weights for Girls 18 Years of Age*

Height (with flat heels)		Weight (in indoor clothing)†		
		Small frame	Medium frame	Large frame
Feet	Inches			
4	10	98-106	105-113	112-122
4	11	100-108	107-115	114-124
5	0	103-111	110-118	117-128
5	1	106-114	113-121	120-131
5	2	109-118	117-125	124-135
5	3	112-121	120-128	126-138
5	4	116-125	123-133	131-143
5	5	119-129	127-137	135-147
5	6	122-132	130-140	138-151

*Adapted from tables prepared by the Metropolitan Life Insurance Company.

†An allowance of 4 pounds is made for a woman's clothing.

Height	Weight (in indoor clothing)		
(with flat heels)	Small frame	Medium frame	Large frame
Feet Inches			
5 7	126-136	134-144	142-155
5 8	129-140	138-148	145-159
5 9	132-143	141-151	148-162

Desirable Weights for Women*
(25 and over)

Height	Weight (in indoor clothing)†		
(with 2-inch heels)	Small frame	Medium frame	Large frame
Feet Inches			
4 10	92-98	96-107	104-119
4 11	94-101	98-110	106-122
5 0	96-104	101-113	109-125
5 1	99-107	104-116	112-128
5 2	102-110	107-119	115-131
5 3	105-113	110-122	118-134
5 4	108-116	113-126	121-138
5 5	111-119	116-130	125-142
5 6	114-123	120-135	129-146
5 7	118-127	124-139	133-150
5 8	122-131	128-143	137-154
5 9	126-135	132-147	141-158
5 10	130-140	136-151	145-163
5 11	134-144	140-155	149-168
6 0	138-148	144-159	153-173

*Adapted from tables prepared by the Metropolitan Life Insurance Company.
†An allowance of 4 pounds is made for a woman's clothing.

Your "ideal" weight depends on your individual skeletal frame and the size of your muscles. Although height and weight tables are based on averages of weights for thousands of people of the same age, height, and frame size, they can still give you a general idea of what people of your classification weigh. You can determine your best weight by judging how you look and feel nude, or dressed in clothing which reveals your figure. Weigh yourself once a week, preferably in the morning (when you weigh slightly less), before you dress. Each week (weighing yourself more often might be discouraging) record your weight and your goal on the following chart:

Weight Record

Date	Weight	Goal	Date	Weight	Goal	Date	Weight	Goal
——	——	——	——	——	——	——	——	——
——	——	——	——	——	——	——	——	——
——	——	——	——	——	——	——	——	——
——	——	——	——	——	——	——	——	——
——	——	——	——	——	——	——	——	——

SET YOUR FIGURE GOALS AND REACH THEM

Anyone can have a healthier and more attractive body if she wants it enough to work for it. Begin by setting a realistic goal for 6 months; then establish more easily reached weekly goals to attain along the way. For example, if your goal is to lose 20 pounds in 6 months spread the total amount of weight loss you desire over monthly periods, and work for a pre-determined number of pounds to be lost each week.

NUTRITION AND TOTAL FITNESS   5

You can lose weight only by eating fewer calories than you burn through daily physical activity (your body will begin to burn its stored fat to supplement the loss). When you supply your body with just enough calories to meet its demands, your weight will remain constant. If you eat more than your body can burn the excess is stored in the form of fat, which will accumulate first around the stomach, hips, upper arms, and chin. Once your weight is within the correct range (as shown on the charts on pages 18–19, chapter 4), you should maintain that level throughout your life. Most people become less active as they grow older. And, although your body will require less food, you will probably continue to eat the same amount as you did when younger. As a result, your body will lose its shape and efficiency. You must *determine* to eat less, to be more active, and maintain your resolve.

How to Gain Weight

Exercise and a high caloric diet can help the underweight person gain weight and improve her figure, since exercise increases muscle size, which adds weight and shape to the body. To gain weight you need from 200 to 500 calories daily in excess of body needs. It is best to gain steadily and slowly, adding from 1 to 2 pounds a week, until you reach the weight normal for your body type, age, and height.

To gain weight sensibly:

1. Include liberal amounts of the concentrated fuel foods (fats, sugars, and starches) in your daily diet: butter or margarine, cream, salad dressings, bacon, cereals, bread, sugar, rich soups, and meats marbled with fat. (Fats produce 2¼ times more calories than an equivalent amount of carbohydrates or proteins.)

2. Eat more each meal and eat more often. For snacks between meals have malted milk shakes, ice cream, and sweets.

3. Drink a glass of milk with each meal.

4. Have a snack before bed and increase the number of your sleeping hours and daily resting time.

5. Increase your intake of high protein foods (milk, eggs, cheese, and meat).

Exercise moderately every day.

HOW MANY CALORIES DO YOU NEED DAILY?

The calorie, the amount of heat needed to raise 1 kilogram (2.2 pounds) of water 1 degree Fahrenheit — is the key to weight control. To "count your calories," record the calorie value of the food you eat daily. (See pp. 00, 00, and 00 for lists of high and low calorie foods.)

Each calorie packs a tremendous amount of energy! One food calorie is equivalent in mechanical energy to 1.54 foot tons (the energy required to lift a ton of weight 1.54 feet). A glass of milk (150 calories) could raise 10 men, each weighing 200 pounds, about 230 feet.[8] Some foods are much higher in calorie content than others. For example, one normal serving of cabbage is only 5 calories, whereas 10 potato chips 2 inches in diameter contain 110 calories; one wedge of honeydew melon has only 59 calories, and one regular size cola drink between 84 and 100 calories.

To discover how many calories you need, use the following illustration:

A moderately active woman of medium frame who is 5 feet 5 inches tall should weigh about 134 pounds. If she weighs more, she can calculate her daily calorie quota for losing one pound a week in the following way:

(1) She finds her normal daily requirement: 134 (her present weight) multiplied by 15 (average number of calories burned per day per pound of body weight) = 2010 (her daily requirement for maintaining her present weight).

(2) She subtracts 500 calories (lowering total intake of calories to below minimum requirement for maintaining weight).

(3) 1510 calories is her daily quota for reducing.[9]

Since it takes a deficiency of 3500 calories (the number of calories contained in each pound of fat) to lose one pound of fat, reducing food intake 500 calories daily will cause one to lose one pound in one week, 4.3 pounds in one month, and nearly 13 pounds in 90 days. Although this weekly loss seems slight, it becomes significant over several months. All diets below 1000 calories per day should be undertaken only under a physician's supervision.

[8]Fred Hein and Dana Farnsworth, *Living*, 4th Edition (Dallas: Scott, Foresman and Company), 1965, p. 79.

[9]American Institute of Baking, *Eat and Grow Slim*, by permission.

Most high school and college girls require a daily intake of approximately 2300 calories, depending on how active they are and their height and weight. The secret of healthful eating is a balanced diet. Every day you need foods from each of the four basic food groups shown below:

DAILY FOOD GUIDE*
THE BASIC FOUR FOR THE ENTIRE FAMILY

GROUPS	*DAILY AMOUNTS*
MILK GROUP Milk (whole, skim, evaporated; instant non-fat dry; buttermilk), with cheese and ice cream as alternates	Adults: 2 cups Children: 3-4 cups *For calcium:* 1 oz. American cheese equals $\frac{3}{4}$ cup milk $\frac{1}{2}$ cup cottage cheese equals $\frac{1}{3}$ cup milk $\frac{1}{2}$ cup ice cream equals $\frac{1}{4}$ cup milk
MEAT GROUP Meat, poultry, fish, eggs—with dry beans, dry peas and nuts as alternates	2 or more servings. Count as a serving: 2 to 3 ounces of lean cooked meat, poultry or fish; 2 eggs; 1 cup cooked dried beans; 4 tablespoons of peanut butter
VEGETABLE-FRUIT GROUP	4 or more servings. Include: a citrus fruit or other Vitamin C-rich fruit or vegetable daily. A dark leafy green or deep yellow vegetable for Vitamin A at least every other day. Other fruits and vegetables—including potatoes—at least 2 or 3 servings daily. Count as a serving: $\frac{1}{2}$ cup of vegetable or fruit.
BREAD-CEREAL GROUP	4 or more servings. Whole grain or enriched. Count as a serving: 1 slice of bread, 1 ounce ready-to-eat cereal; $\frac{1}{2}$ to $\frac{3}{4}$ cup cooked cereal, noodles, rice, etc.

Note: Fats, oils and sugars can be combined with many foods to enhance flavor, but should be used sparingly. Although water is not a nutrient, it is essential to proper body functioning.

*Reproduced by permission of the National Dairy Council, Chicago, Illinois.

For weight loss to be permanent, it should be slow and steady. Increased physical activity alone will not take pounds off. Steinhaus, a leading physiologist, discovered that to lose a single pound of weight one would have to walk 44 miles or run 129 separate 100-yard dashes in 10 seconds each. Diet or reducing pills are extremely dangerous unless taken under a reputable doctor's orders. Crash diets are almost worthless, for they have little lasting effect. Human beings respond better to pleasure and gratification than to discipline and self-denial. When we deny ourselves food during a crash diet program, we often reward ourselves for reaching the desired weight by eating, often more voraciously than before. Frederick Stare, an authority on weight loss and nutrition, calls most reducing diets foolish, for many promised shortcuts to weight loss have no scientific basis, and some are very dangerous. He has found that those who undertake severe crash diets soon regain their lost weight and tend to gain even more than before.

> Weight loss depends on negative caloric balance, and not specifically on carbohydrate, protein, or fat, except as they contribute to the total calories of the diet. Studies in which obese women consumed varying proportions of fat, carbohydrate or protein have reported no relationship between weight loss and the composition of the diet eaten when total caloric levels were similar.[10]

Remember, there is only one way to become healthier, trimmer, and more attractive — eat less, eat well-balanced meals, and exercise more. Remember, too, that your initial weight loss will be rapid — due largely to loss of water from body tissues. Next, like most people, you will reach a plateau when you stop losing weight, even though you are following the same activity patterns and dietary habits. If you take your measurements, you will find that your body has begun redistributing fat and you are beginning to look trim. With this in mind, don't lose faith in the diet, or the physical activity. It is as important to shift weight and become trim as it is to shed pounds.

[10]Frederick Stare, M.D., "Diet Shortcuts Will Lead To Weight-Loss Dead End" (*The Dallas Morning News,* Thursday, April 22, 1971), p. 2E.

The Calories You Use Per Hour Per Single Pound of Your Weight*

Activity	Calories Used†
Sleeping	.43
Awake, motionless	.50
Just sitting	.65
Standing relaxed	.69
Hand sewing	.72
Typewriting rapidly	.91
Ironing, dishwashing	.93
Light exercise	1.10
Walking slowly	1.30
Carpentry	1.56
"Active" exercise	1.88
Walking downstairs	2.36
"Severe" exercise	2.92
Swimming	3.25
Running	3.70
"Very severe" exercise	3.90
Walking fast (5.3 mph)	4.22
Walking upstairs	7.18

*From *A New Figure in 30 Days* (New York: Dell Publishing Co., Dell Purse Book No. 6324), 1970.

†Multiply by your weight to find out how much energy you use.

HOW TO STAY TRIM FOREVER

You can *stay* slim and trim forever if you:

1. Eat less, but be sure that you eat three well-balanced meals every day.

2. Have a light breakfast of 200 to 300 calories. (This will help you eat less for lunch and dinner.)

3. Do not eat fried foods if you can help it and never eat the fat of meat. (Remember the 3B's of weight loss and food preparation — bake, broil, or boil!)

4. Allow yourself an occasional spree, but be sure to eat sparingly the next day. Remember the pleasure-pain theory of human behavior and that

we all seek the former over the latter. The results of changed eating habits will give you more pleasure than a crash diet, which is undeniably painful.

5. Always stop eating before you feel full.

6. Eat those foods slowly that take time and have a low caloric count.

7. Use pleasing color in food selection (yellow and green vegetables are highest in vitamin content) and serve portions in smaller dishes. (These simple deceptions work wonders.)

8. Use salt sparingly; it causes the body to· retain water, which slows circulation and makes one feel sluggish.

9. Avoid second helpings of all foods but those with fewer than 100 calories.

10. Drink diet soft drinks; remember that alcoholic drinks are loaded with calories.

11. Keep busy. When you have an urge to snack do something active and move physically away from that temptation.

12. Start your meals with low calorie appetizers, such as clear broths or vegetable soups, fruit or vegetable juices. (Liquids help fill you up.)

13. Drink skim milk and use it in cooking.

14. Be on the lookout for fat people on the bus, walking down the street, or in magazine pictures. Vow never to let yourself become as fat and unattractive.

15. Have a snapshot taken of you in a tight dress or in a bathing suit. Look at it often. Have other pictures taken periodically for comparison.

16. Weigh yourself once a week. Do not get discouraged if, after your first weight loss (which is largely water) it is harder to keep losing. Remember that the most permanent type of weight loss is a gradual shedding of 1 to 2 pounds weekly.

17. Avoid sugar-sweetened and doughy foods such as candy, cola, cookies, doughnuts, gelatin desserts, jelly, pancakes, pies, sweet rolls, and waffles. Use only noncaloric sweeteners as you learn to like unsweetened foods. Avoid honey or molasses as sweeteners.

18. Keep busy to take your mind off food and keep imagining how

lovely you will look when you reach your figure goal. Pamper yourself by wearing your favorite perfume more often, having your hair done more frequently, and buying new things for your room.

19. Fall in love.

FOODS AND DRINKS THAT ADD UNNECESSARY CALORIES

Make up your mind not to snack between meals. If you find the desire for snacks the most difficult part of your newly forming eating habits, you will be amazed how chewing sugarless gum will help you avoid this dieter's trap.

Parties undo in a short time what has been painstakingly accomplished. Weight control is a habit easily broken.

When partying and dining out, remember to:

Select the foods at a buffet or from a menu that are the lowest in calories (lean meats, green or yellow vegetables, salads without dressing).

Have a glass of orange juice or skim milk before leaving home.

Select low calorie soft drinks; stay away from calorie-loaded dips, nuts, and other tidbits.

When you go to a party move around often and keep yourself farthest away from the refreshments. Develop your conversational skills.

The following chart will warn you of foods high in calories and low in food value.

*Foods that Contribute Little More Than Calories to the Diet**

Food	Amount	Calories
Alcoholic beverages:		
Beer	12-ounce can	170
Hard liquor (70-100 proof)	1½ ounces (1 jigger)	100-145
Wine:		
light table wines	3 ounces	75
sherry, port	3 ounces	130

*Source: N.Y. State College of Home Economics, Cornell University. Reproduced by permission.

Cake, angel or sponge, unfrosted	2″ section of an 8″ cake	110
Cake, shortened, unfrosted	2″ x 3″ x 1½″	180
Candy or frosting	1 ounce	100-150
Carbonated beverages	8 ounces	105
Cookies:		
brownie or chocolate chip	1 average size	65
homemade drop	1, 2″ diameter	40
Crackers: saltine or other types	1	15
Jam or jelly	1 tablespoon	50
Olives	1 medium large	12
Pie	⅐ of a 9″ pie	300-350
Potato chips	10, 2″ diameter	110
Potatoes, french fried	1 serving	275
Puddings:		
cornstarch, tapioca,		
custard	½ cup	135-175
Salad dressings:		
French	1 tablespoon	50
mayonnaise	1 tablespoon	100
Sherbet	½ cup	95-130
Soup: condensed commercial varieties		
cream soups (diluted with milk)	1 cup	160
stock soups (diluted with water)	1 cup	65

The Yo-Yo Weight Syndrome.   Those who go on crash diets, lose some weight and gain it back again are victims of the Yo-Yo Weight Syndrome, the weight-up-weight-down pattern. According to medical experts studying obesity, the yo-yo syndrome dieter whose weight seesaws greatly needs medical help.[11] A study involving 1,000 subjects, including normal weight people as a control group, concluded that if one is 20 percent above or below her ideal weight, she has potentially serious metabolic problems, possibly caused by over- or undereating, and should consult a physician.

Obesity – A Health Hazard.   There is medical evidence that obesity is directly related to heart disease, diabetes, arthritis, gout, high blood pressure, kidney disease, high cholesterol level, hernia, thyroid disease, colitis, and peptic ulcers. But only 5 percent of obesity is due to physiological reasons. Obesity shortens life expectancy; it is a self-imposed premature death sentence resulting from over indulgence in food. Every excess pound of fat requires about 4,500 feet of new blood vessels and the expansion of capillaries. Because the heart has to work harder, it breaks

[11]James Conniff, "A Medical Breakthrough" *(Ladies Home Journal,* April 1968), pp. 84-87.

down faster, and so do the other internal organs. The early mortality rate for fat people between the ages of 20 and 65 averages 15 percent higher than for people of normal weight.[12]

Foods with Few or No Calories

	Calories
Asparagus (6 spears)	21
Bouillon (1 cube)	2
Broccoli ($\frac{1}{2}$ cup)	22
Cabbage ($\frac{1}{2}$ cup)	12
Cantaloupe ($\frac{1}{2}$ cup diced)	15
Carrots (1 medium)	21
Cauliflower ($\frac{1}{2}$ cup cooked)	15
Celery (1 stalk)	5
Celery salt	0
Coffee (no cream or sugar)	0
Cucumbers (6 slices)	6
Green beans ($\frac{1}{2}$ cup cooked)	13
Green peppers (1)	15
Lemon juice (1 tablespoon)	4
Lettuce (2 large or 4 small leaves)	5
Mushrooms ($\frac{1}{2}$ cup)	13
Parsley (1 tablespoon chopped)	1
Rhubarb (1 cup, unsweetened)	19
Sauerkraut ($\frac{1}{2}$ cup)	15
Spinach (1 cup raw)	10
Tomatoes (2 slices)	15
Turnips ($\frac{1}{2}$ cup cooked)	21
Water chestnuts (4)	17
Zucchini ($\frac{1}{2}$ cup cooked)	18

Foods with 50 Calories

1 large tomato	4 potato chips
2 cucumbers	5 wheat crackers
1 onion	5 dried apricot halves
1 head of lettuce	1 slice French bread
1 small ear of corn	1 thin slice wheat bread
1 artichoke	1 cup cooked broccoli
1 strip of bacon	1 cup cooked cabbage
1 buckwheat pancake	$1\frac{1}{2}$ tbs. gravy
1 cup strawberries	2 sticks chewing gum
1 large peach	1 tortilla
1 average slice of watermelon	1 chocolate cookie
1 tbs. cream cheese	2 graham crackers
3 medium oysters	1 macaroon
3 apricots	3 small carrots

[12] Andrew Williams, *You Can Reduce* (New York: Hearthside Press, 1962), p. 16.

Foods with 100 Calories

<table>
<tr><td>

1 scrambled egg
1 medium crab
½ chicken breast
1 ounce roast lamb
1 ounce roast pork
2 ounces roast chicken
1 slice cheese
1 shredded wheat biscuit
1 cup corn flakes
1 soft roll
1 bran muffin
1 baked potato
½ cup macaroni
⅔ cup spaghetti
1 whole small grapefruit
4 large prunes

</td><td>

1 cup canned cherries
1 slice watermelon
1 cup unsweetened applesauce
½ cup canned peaches
1 large glass skim milk
1 large glass buttermilk
1 large glass ginger ale
1 large glass dry wine
1 slice angel food cake
1 tbs. mayonnaise
1 cup orange juice
1 shrimp cocktail
1 cup green peas
1 cup cole slaw
½ cup cottage cheese

</td></tr>
</table>

SLIMNASTIC EXERCISES **6**

YOUR EXERCISE PROGRAM

Set aside 30 minutes each day for your exercise program. Eventually you should exercise for an hour a day at least three times a week. Begin gradually by moving your body rhythmically to music. Hard exercise without warm-up causes sore muscles and you may be discouraged from continuing. Divide each session into easy rhythmic warm-ups combined with deep breathing, and then progress to more strenuous movements to increase your stamina and cardiovascular efficiency.

The best time to exercise depends upon the individual; you might prefer the morning, or at night before going to bed. It is not a matter of *when* you exercise, but of *how often* and *how vigorously* you do it. Only by pushing yourself to do a bit more each time can you build strength and endurance (the principle of overload and adaptation — the body must work against resistance or progressively greater load, whether it be increased repetition, or increased speed). Try to augment the number of exercises you can already do by a few more each day. Wear clothing that permits you to move easily. Stretch shorts and blouses or leotards are better than slacks for free movement. Follow your exercise period with a brisk shower. You might also try exercising with friends — the companionship diverts you from the effort. Deep breathing should be part of your program of vigorous exercise — it increases the lung's capacity, creating a greater oxygen supply for the body. Running out doors is an ideal way for you to discover the difference between normal shallow breathing and deep breathing (which, like increased perspiration, helps rid the body of waste products). The circulatory system, like the muscular system, deteriorates rapidly through inactivity or underuse. Race your motor occasionally — it's healthy.

The *frequency* (every day); *intensity* (exercise with spirit, so that you breathe more deeply and perspire more freely); and *duration* (exercise until you tingle, then start to tire) of your exercise program are most important. Other factors to remember are:

Daily exercise will keep your body toned and flexible and make you feel better.

It is easier to keep a good figure than to achieve or regain one. Ninety days of inactivity can undo 60 days of training.

Exercise should become a routine, like brushing your teeth.

Running, jogging, and swimming are the best overall figure trimmers and calorie burners.

Exercise can help you gain strength and gracefulness.

BODY CONDITIONING EXERCISES

1. *Running*   Run outdoors or run in place 25 strides (count 1 stride each time your right foot touches the ground or floor). Raise your legs high and pump your arms vigorously. Increase to 50, 100, 150, 200, 250 times.

2. *Arm and Leg Lift*   With arms at sides, on 1, swing both arms up, tighten stomach, lift left leg as high as it will go. On 2, bring leg and arms down. Do rapidly 25, 50, 75, 100, 125 times. Repeat using the right leg.

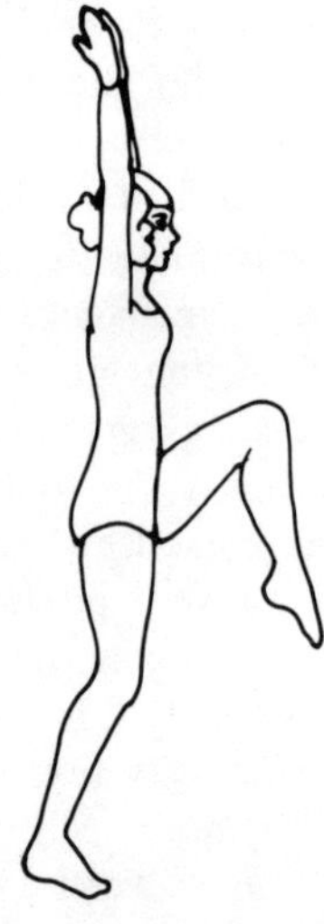

3. *Jumping Jack*   Hands at sides, feet in a wide stride position. On 1, bring feet together and clap hands overhead. On 2, return to the stride position with hands at sides. Repeat rapidly 25, 50, 75, 100, 125 times.

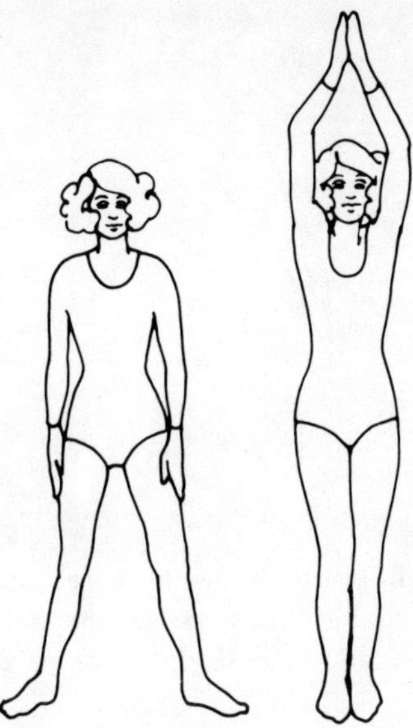

4. *Bent Knees Sit-up*   Lie on your back with knees bent, hands clasped behind head. Have someone hold your feet or anchor them under a heavy chair. On 1, sit up, bend to touch right elbow to left knee; on 2, lie down; 3, sit up, bend to touch left elbow to right knee; 4, lie down. Do 4 to 6 times at first, then gradually increase to 25 times. Do slowly at first, then quickly.

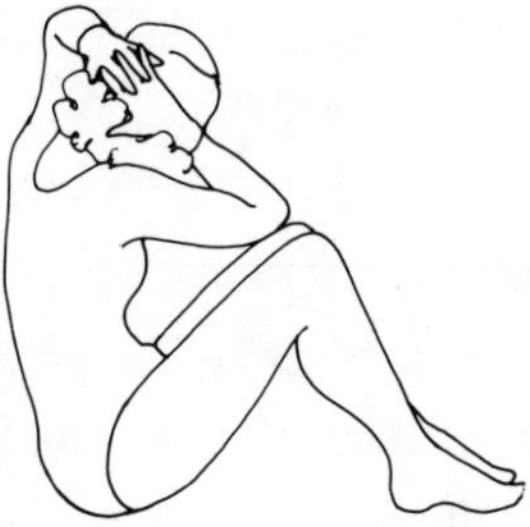

5. *Jump Starts*   In a semi-crouched position, hands at your sides, feet apart, alternate crouching and jumping high with body in full extension. Repeat jump-crouch 4 to 6 times and gradually increase to 10.

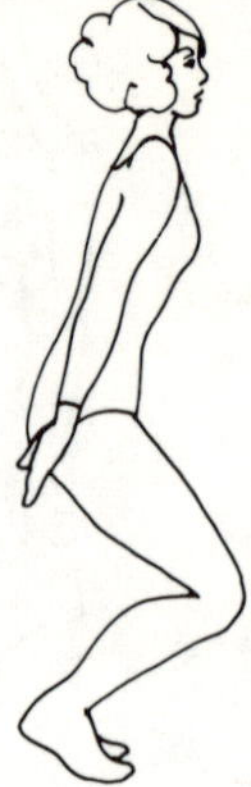

6. *Jumping Rope*   Jump with single rope, stretching arms high. Increase speed, jumping double time to music, then taper off to single time. Jump as long as you can. Try to jump during an entire song.

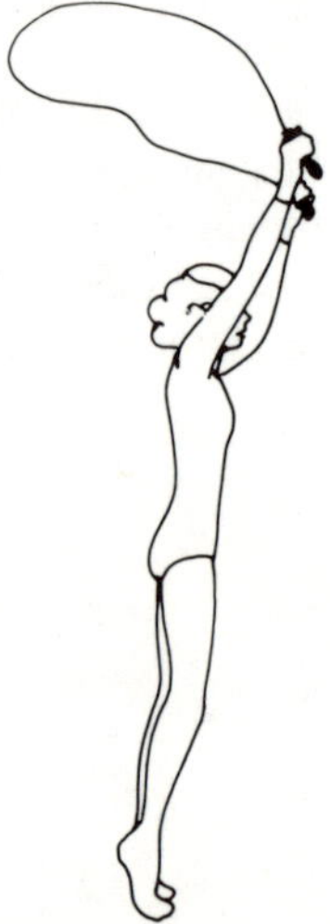

EXERCISES FOR THE WAISTLINE

1. *Hand and Toe Touch*   Arms out to the sides at shoulder level. On 1, swing left leg over and up to touch the right hand (do not lower hand to touch your toes). On 2, return to place. On 3 and 4, repeat movements with right leg. Repeat 10 times.

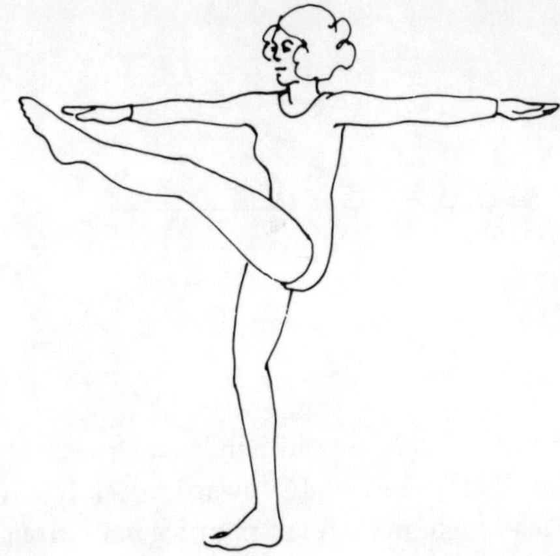

2. *Curl-up*   Lie on your back with fingers laced together behind your neck, legs bent. On 1, curl trunk forward to sitting position, bend to touch left elbow to right, then left, knee. On 2, lie down. Repeat 10 times, alternating knee touches. (Have someone hold your feet or anchor them under heavy furniture at first.)

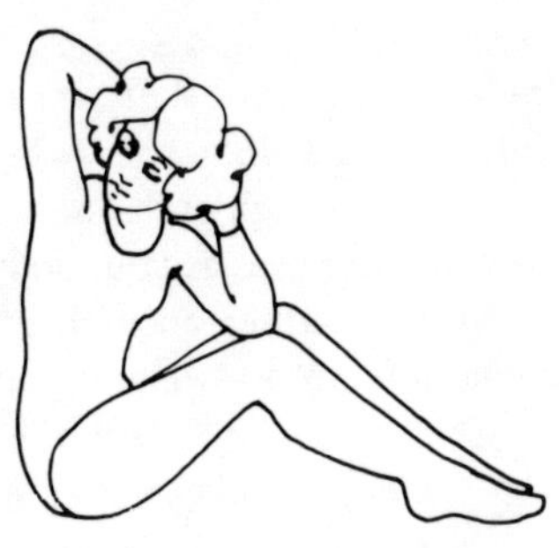

3. *Jackknife*   Lie on your back with body extended. On 1, curl up, extend both arms forward and up, and reach to touch toes, holding your body in a sideways V (jackknife) position. On 2, return to place. Repeat 10 times.

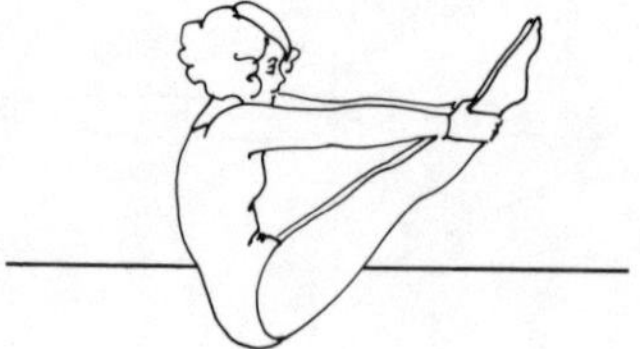

4. *Nose-Knee Kiss*   Kneel on your hands and knees, keeping your torso straight and head up. On 1, curl body toward knees touching nose to right knee. On 2, raise head high and stretch right leg back straight. Do 10 times. Change, bringing left knee to touch your nose, and repeat 10 times.

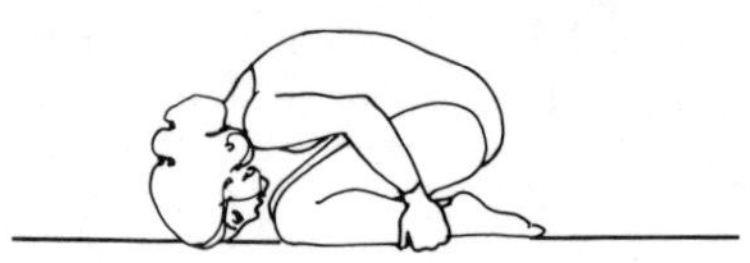

5. *Threading the Needle*   Kneel with left arm bent and palm on floor. On 1, sweep right shoulder to the floor and swing right arm through the arch made by the left arm. On 2, swing right arm out and briskly to the side, following the movement with your eyes as your body twists and straightens. Do 10 times, swinging the arm farther on each sweep in, and thrust out. Reverse position, using your left arm to swing; repeat 10 times.

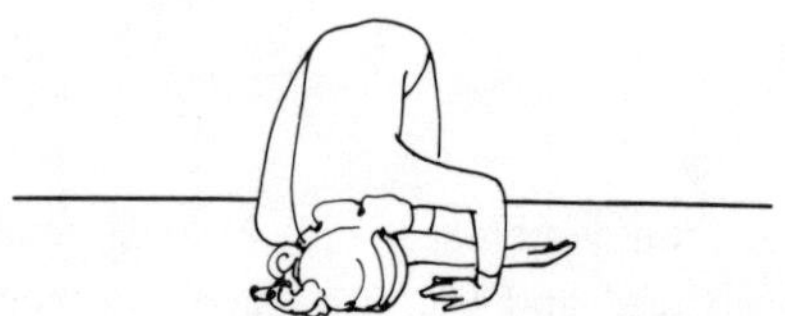

6. *Shoulder Level Hand Kick*   Stand with hands on hips. On 1, raise the right arm to shoulder level, at the same time kick with the left leg, touching the right hand to the raised foot as close to the big toe as you can by rotating your trunk and pelvis. Repeat for 5 counts. Then kick with right leg and touch with left hand for 5 counts. Try to avoid bending from the waist, losing your balance, or bending your supporting leg. Do 25 of these on each leg.

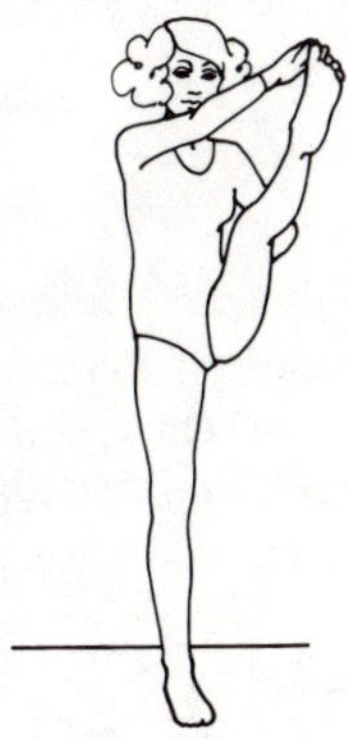

7. *Windmill*   Stand erect, arms held out at shoulder level, feet wide apart. On 1, twist body to side at the waist, touch floor behind right foot with left hand, then return to erect position on 2. On 3, twist and touch behind left foot with right hand. On 4, return to erect position. Repeat 20 times.

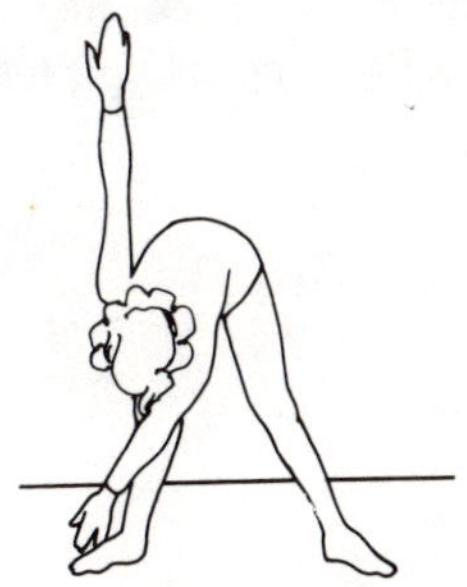

8. *Rocker*   Lying on your stomach, legs bent, curl body back and grasp your ankles, keeping legs far apart. On 1, pull up as far as you can, raising your head, and rocking your body back and forth. On 2, relax; repeat on 3 and 4. Do 10 times.

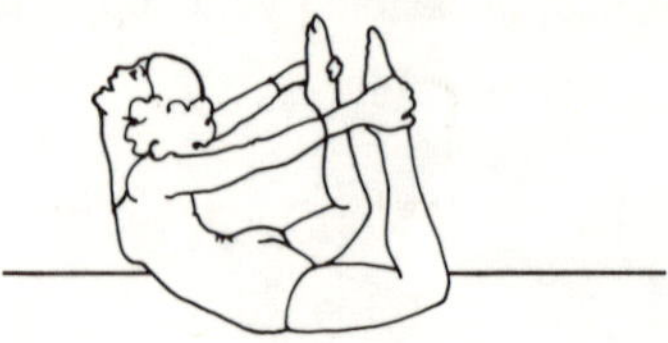

9. *Chair Sit-up*   Lie on your back, with legs, body, and arms fully extended, heels on the edge of a chair. On 1, curl up to touch toes, return to place on 2. Begin gradually and work up to 15 repetitions of this.

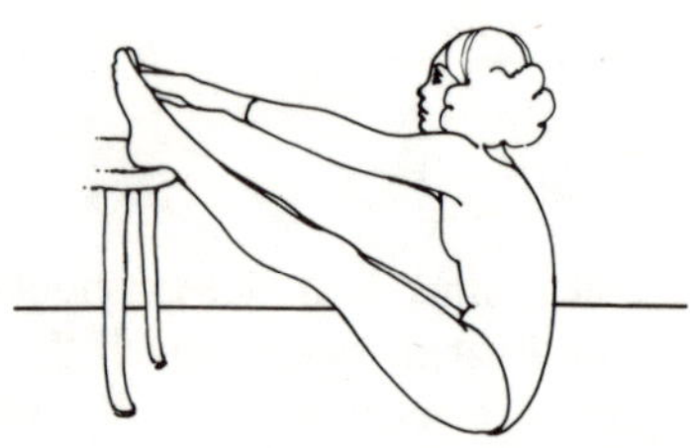

10. *Slow Leg Lift*   Lie on your back, fingers laced behind neck. On 1, flex both legs; on 2, extend legs straight up pointing toes. On 3, lower legs slowly. Do 10 of these.*

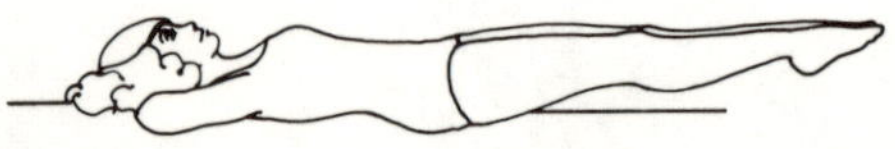

*Many physiologists do not recommend this exercise – keeping the knees locked exerts a reverse pull on the psoas major which can contribute to low back pain or lordosis. Others agree that it is a good exercise if you keep your back in contact with the floor.

11. *Peddle Kick Out*   Sit with legs fully extended on the floor. On 1, lean back halfway, extend arms forward, raise knees, and mimic peddling a bicycle. On 2, return to place. On 3, lean back, raise legs with body in a V position with arms, hands, legs, and toes in full extension. Work up to 10 of these.

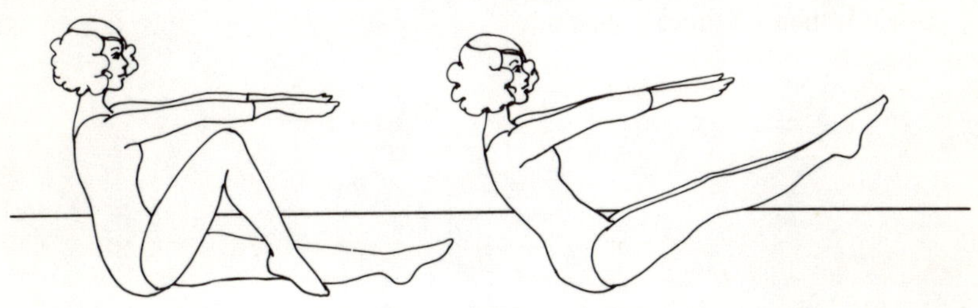

12. *Backbend Toe Touch*   Stand erect. On 1, bend knees slightly, arch back, stretch arms down and behind you. On 2, straighten legs and reach up with arms and body, standing on tip toes. On 3, bend forward and touch your toes. On 4, return to erect position.

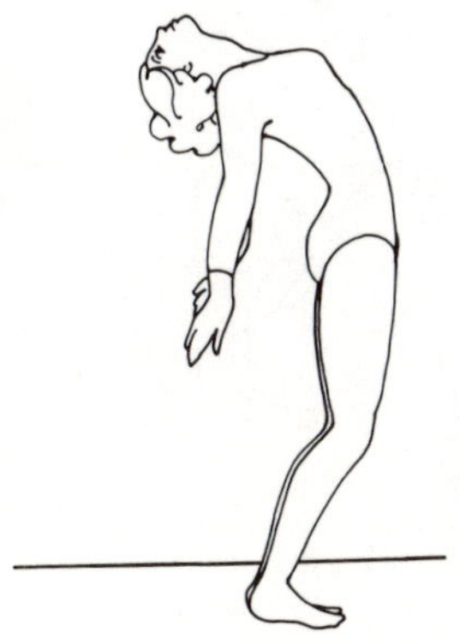

EXERCISES FOR THE HIPS AND THIGHS

1. *Hip Walk*   Sit erect with legs forward and straight, arms forward at shoulder level. On 1, shift weight to left hip and move right hip forward. On 2, shift weight to right hip and move left hip forward. Swing your arms vigorously up and down with each movement. Move quickly 10 times forward, then 10 times backward.

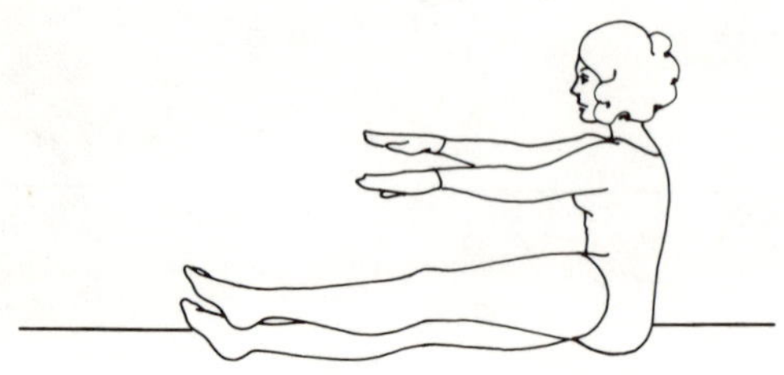

2. *Knee Grasp and Pull*   Stand erect. On 1, bend left leg and pull to your chest. On 2, return foot to floor. Repeat knee grasp and pull with right leg on counts of 3 and 4. Do 15 times for each leg.

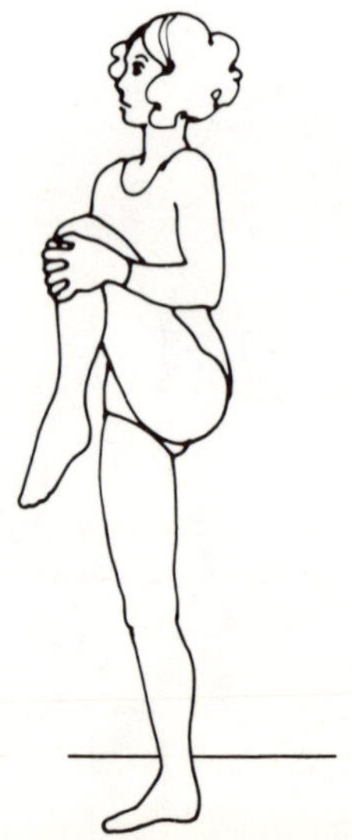

3. *Prone Leg Circle*   Lie on stomach with weight on your forearms and legs fully extended. On 1, raise left leg, keeping knee straight, and circle it 10 times counterclockwise, then 10 times clockwise. On 2, lower it to floor. Repeat with right leg on 3 and 4. As you rotate each leg, try to make each circle larger.

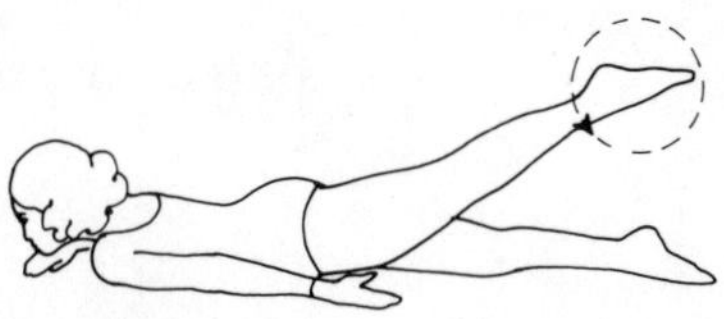

4. *Leg Whips*   Lie on your left side, head resting on extended left arm, legs together and fully extended. For 10 counts, move your right leg sharply up and down. On 11, bend leg and pull it to your chest with your right hand. On 12, release leg and kick backward behind body. Then turn body and repeat with left leg. (Do this for one full band of a long playing record.)

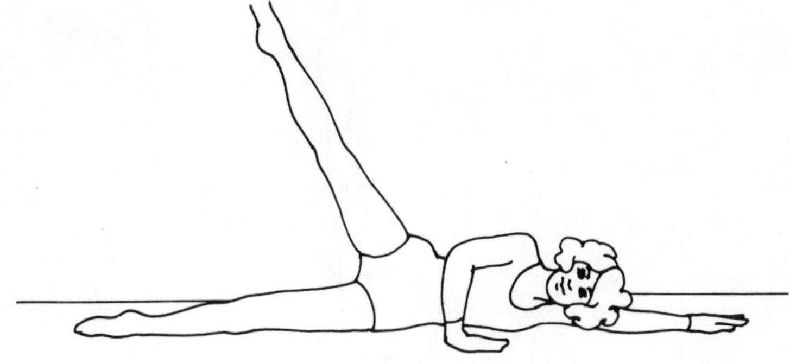

5. *Bicycle Ride*   Lie on your back, with upper arms and elbows on floor, prop hips up with hands, raise body into the air, and peddle legs in time to music. Bring legs together and touch toes on the floor behind your head, then slowly return to resting position.

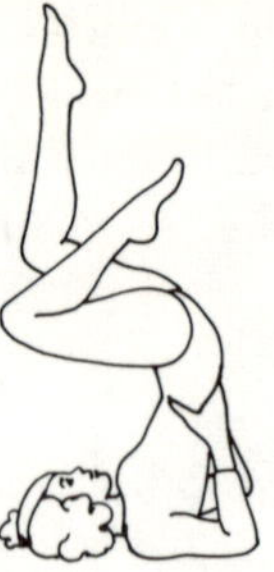

6. *Bench Step*   Stand in front of a chair or bench approximately 14 inches high. Step onto the chair with your right foot, then bring up left foot. Lower right foot to the floor, then lower left foot. Repeat for one minute, eventually increasing to three minutes or more.

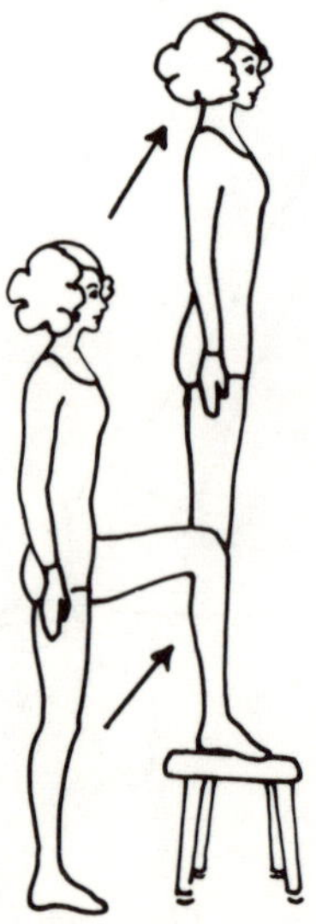

7. *Squat Jumps*   Stand erect with arms at sides. On 1, rise to tip toes. On 2, bend knees (keeping them together) and extend arms forward. On 3, jump high, stretching arms, legs, and feet. On 4, return to place. Repeat 10 times or more.

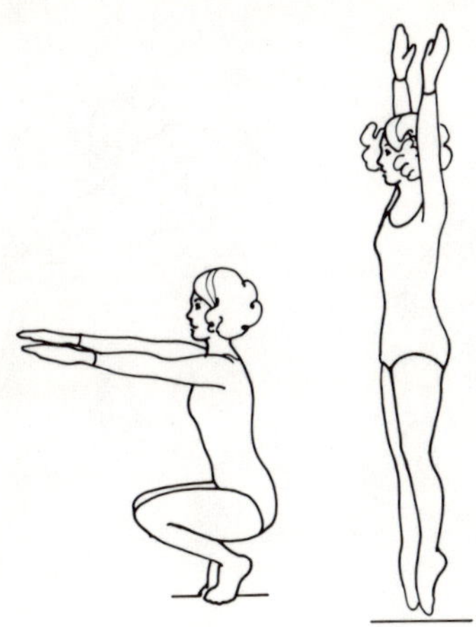

8. *Leg Jumping Jack*   Crouch on hands and toes, with left leg bent under body and right leg back and straight. On 1, reverse feet, so that right leg is bent and left leg is extended behind. Alternate feet and increase speed. Increase endurance gradually to 20 times.

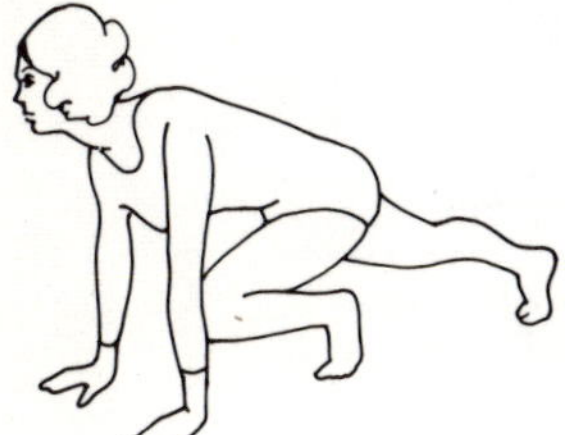

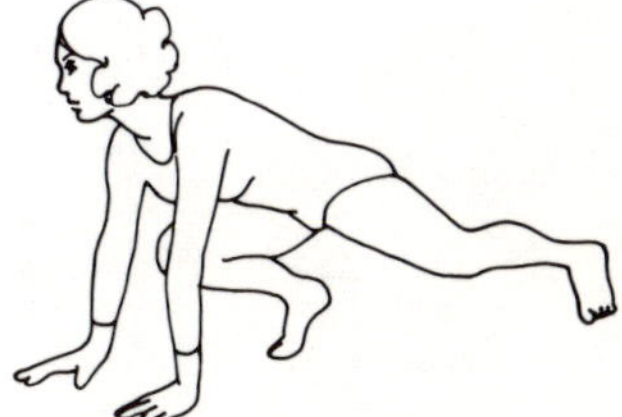

9. *Leg Lock*   Bend body forward and place both hands on the back of a chair. On 1, bend left leg and place it on the chair between your hands. On 2, keeping right knee locked, straighten left leg. On 3, reverse positions and raise flexed right leg to the chairback, then straighten it. Repeat, alternating legs.

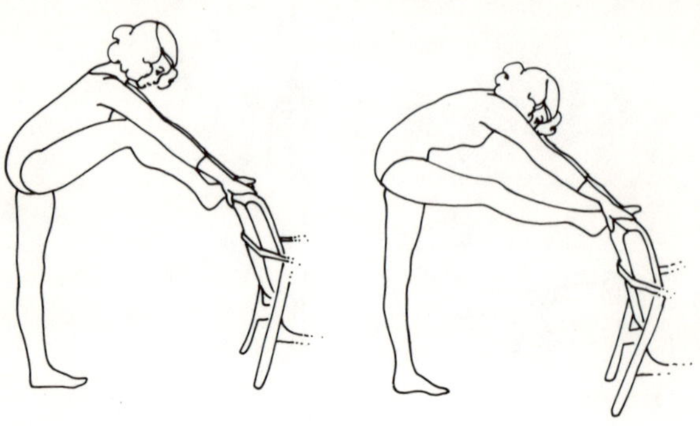

10. *Crossed Leg Push*   Sit cross-legged. On counts 1 to 10, grasp knees and move legs up and down rapidly with your hands. Relax; repeat 15 times.

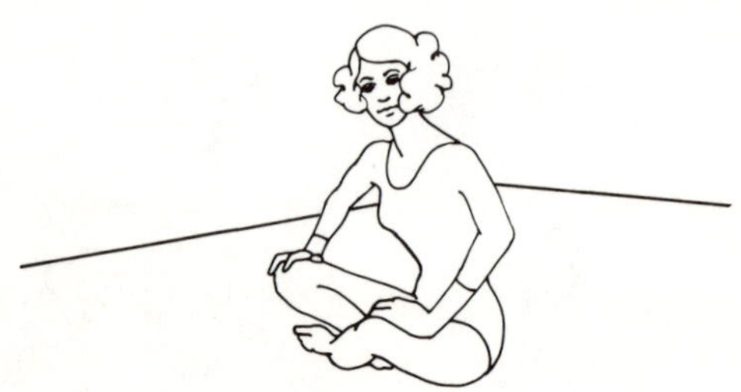

11. *Bent Leg Kick Out*   Sit on the floor, leaning back on your hands, legs extended. On 1, bend knees and raise them together with toes pointed, bringing them as close to your bust as you can. On 2, lean back farther and extend legs (still held together with toes pointed). Repeat 15 times. As you gain strength, increase to 25 times. Then do the exercise without supporting your body as you lean back, first 10 times, then 20 times.

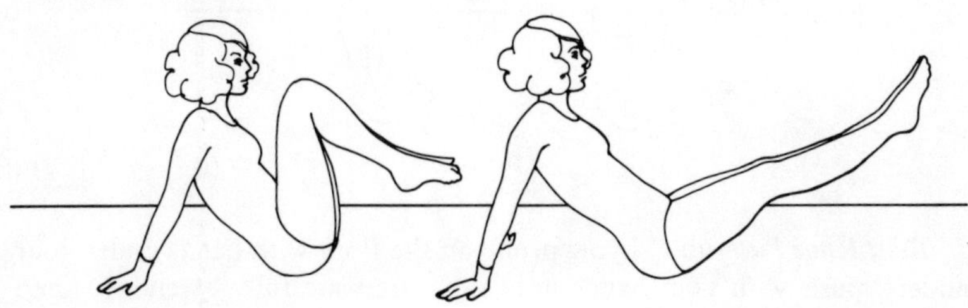

12. *Flutter Kick and Pitty-Pat*   Lie on floor with body straight. On 1, raise legs together with toes pointed and flutter kick (moving legs up and down rapidly) 20 times, at the same time spanking your hips. Then relax. Repeat until you can do this 30 times without resting. (The spanking motion will help increase circulation and break down fat deposits.)

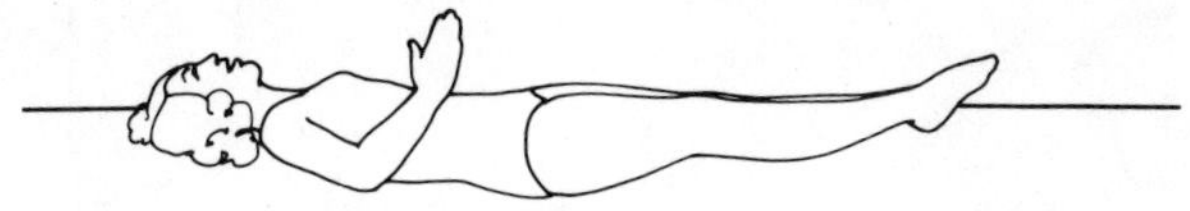

EXERCISES FOR THE BUST, CHEST, AND ARMS

1. *Swan Dive*   Stand with your feet apart. Bend from the hips, keeping back straight. On 1, raise arms behind you and move in opposing circles 10 times. On 2, repeat with arms in front. On 3, behind; 4, in front; 5, relax.

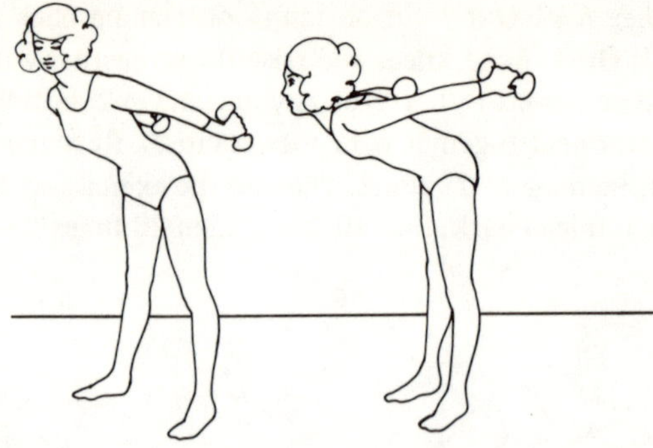

2. *Bent Knee Push-up*   Lying prone on the floor with hands under your shoulders, push with your hands until your arms are fully extended. Keep your body in a straight line from knees to head. Return to original position, keeping body straight. Repeat 10 times and gradually increase.

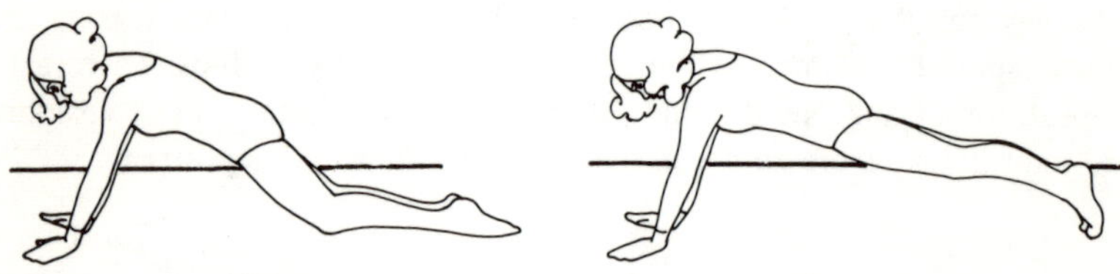

3. *Press*   Stand erect. Clasp hands in front close to your body, right over left. Press your hands against each other as hard as you can, tightening stomach and buttocks muscles. Repeat, clasping hands left over right. Repeat 5 times.

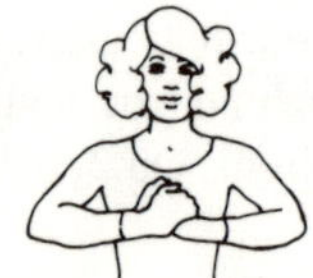

4. *Pullover*   Lie on your back. Hold books, bricks, or other heavy objects in each hand, arms extended behind your head. Point toes, tighten stomach muscles, keep body taut. On 1, lift objects over head and down to your sides, elbows stiff. On 2, return arms behind head. Repeat 15 times. (For variation, hold arms extended sideways. On 1, raise arms straight up. On 2, return to place. Repeat 15 times.)

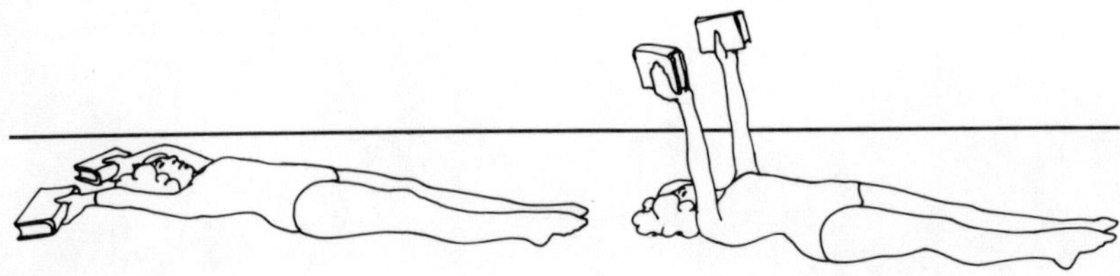

5. *Rope or Wand Stretcher*   Stand straight with feet together. Hold a thin rope, wand, or straight stick above your head with your arms stretched far apart. On 1, bend to the side, trying to touch your left hand to your knees and stretching your right hand over your head. On 2, return to place. On 3, repeat on the right side. Repeat 15 times.

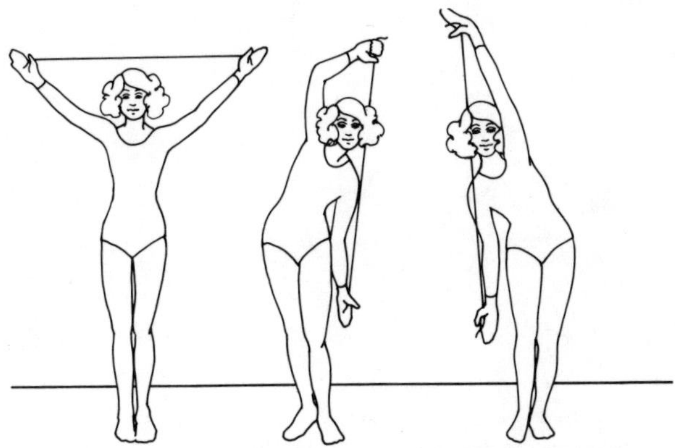

EXERCISES FOR THE FEET AND ANKLES

1. *Alphabet*   Sit on a chair with one leg crossed over the other. Using the top leg, with the toes pointed, write the letters of the alphabet from A to M. Recross your legs and continue writing the alphabet with the other foot. Next, standing on your left foot write the entire alphabet with your right foot, keeping your balance; repeat using the left foot.

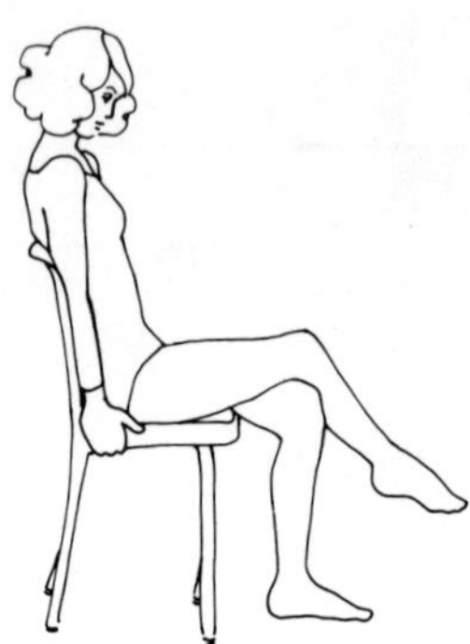

2. *Book Toe-Curl*   Curl your toes over a telephone directory, standing tall with heels on the floor. Raise and lower your body slowly. Repeat 10 times.

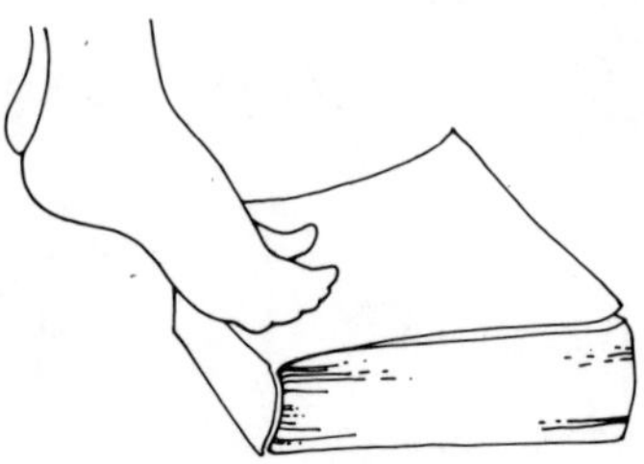

3. *Heel-Toe Lift*   Standing with feet apart, rise to your toes and stretch your entire body as high as you can; on 2, relax with feet flat on the floor. On 3, balance on your heels; on 4, return to place. Repeat 20 times.

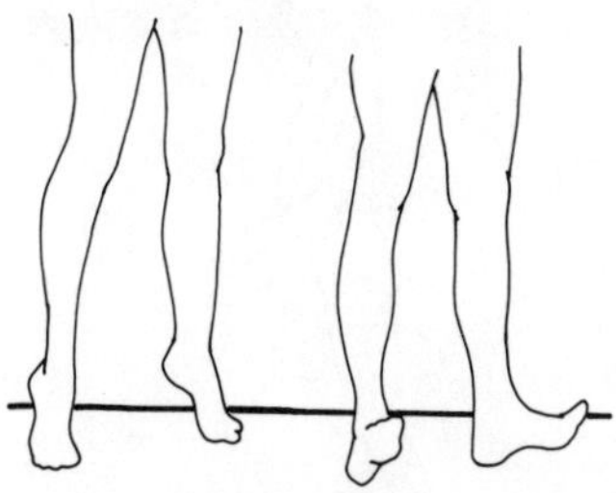

4. *Foot-Stick Press*   Sitting on the floor, and holding a wand, stick, or taut thin rope in front of you with both hands, draw your left knee forward to your chest. On 1, press the ball of your left foot firmly against the stick as you pull it toward your body; on 2, relax. On 3 and 4, repeat with your right foot. Alternating feet, repeat 20 times for each leg.

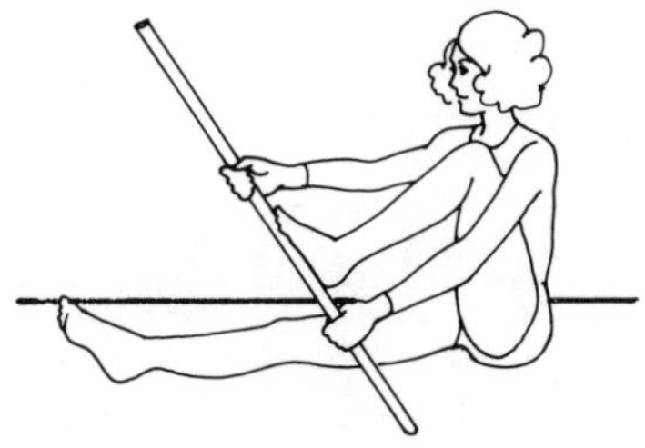

5. *Tiptoe Upstairs Walk*   Keeping your body straight, walk up stairs on tiptoe without touching heel to stairs. Relax when you reach the top. Using railing for balance, tiptoe backward down the staircase.

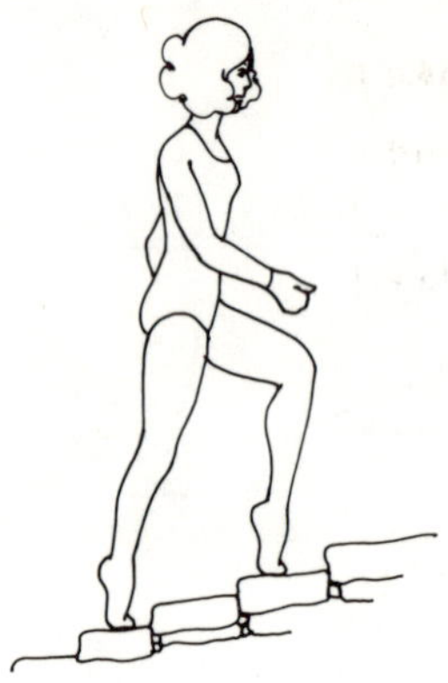

EXERCISES FOR POSTURE IMPROVEMENT

1. *Chair Sit and Arm Fling*   (Strengthens back muscles.) Sit in a chair with arms out to the sides at shoulder level, and legs apart. For two counts bend and touch alternate toes first with your right arm, then the left, each time returning to a sitting position. On 3 return to place. Repeat 20 times.

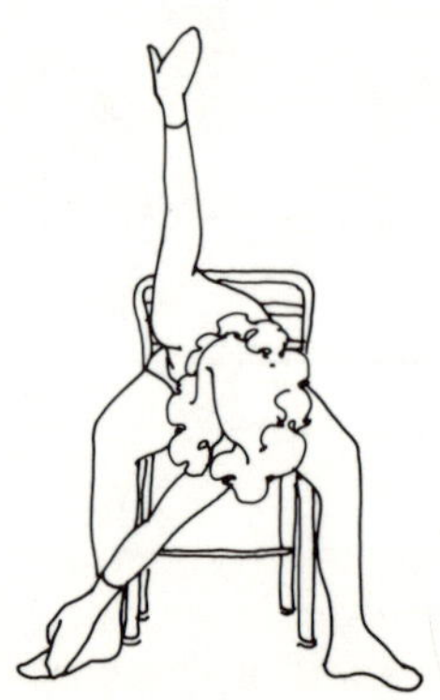

2. *Arm-Wall Slide*   (Strengthens upper body and back muscles.) Sit cross-legged with arms raised above the head, back and arms against the wall. For 4 counts, lower arms gradually until your hands are parallel with your head. Keep your back pressed hard against the wall, and raise arms slowly to overhead position for another four counts. Repeat 15 times.

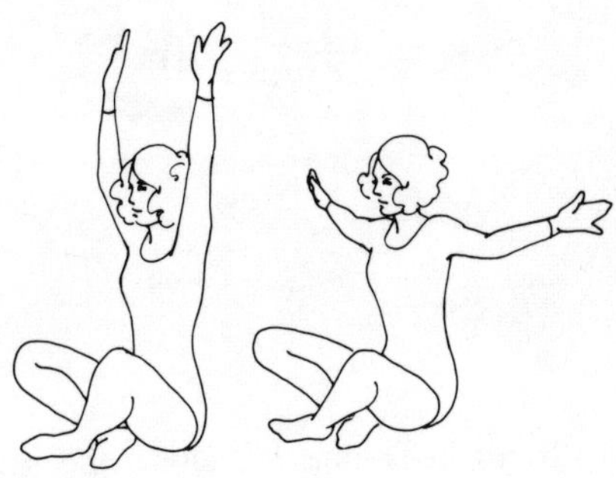

3. *Knee to Nose*   (Strengthens upper body muscles.) Lie on your back with body extended. On 1, bend left leg and raise head and upper body to touch nose to left knee. On 2, lie down. Then repeat exercise with right leg.

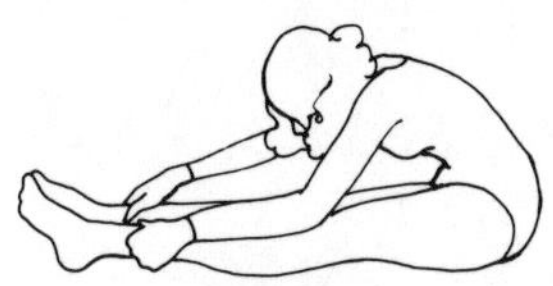

4. *Go Around*   (Strengthens lower back muscles and promotes flexibility.) Sit with legs spread far apart, soles of feet touching partner's, and grasp hands. Lean backward for 4 counts; pulling partner gently toward

you, twist your bodies and move your arms around in a circle. Relax. Then partner pulls you forward and around for 4 counts. Increase to 10 times.

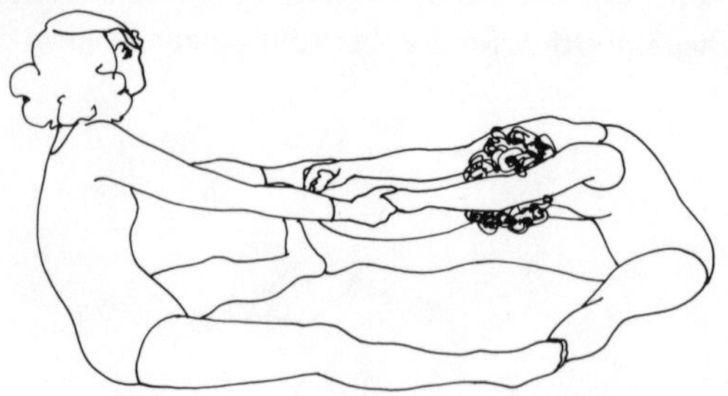

5. *Trunk Bob*   (Strengthens muscles along the spine and promotes flexibility.) Stand with your feet apart, knees locked. Bend forward to touch the floor in front of your right foot; then in front; next behind you, reaching back as far as you can; finally, in front of your left foot. Repeat 10 times. Once you can touch your fingertips to the floor, strive to touch your palms to it.

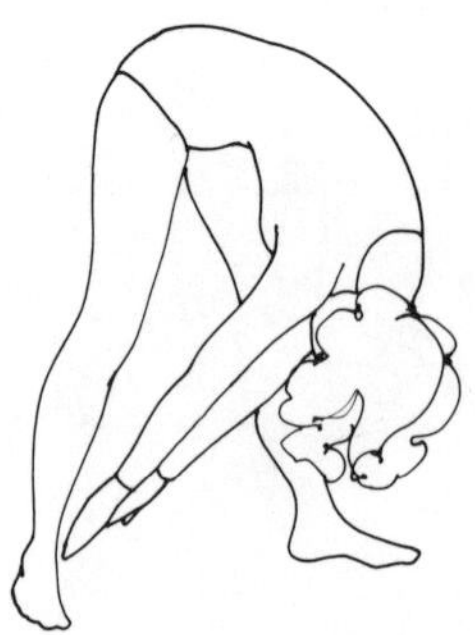

YOGA RELAXATION EXERCISES

1. *Yoga Plow*   Lie on the floor on your back with arms beside your

body. Inhale deeply and exhale slowly as you raise your legs up and over your head, touching your toes on the floor behind your head. Hold your breath for 10 slow counts in this position. Exhale slowly while you bring your legs back down to the floor.

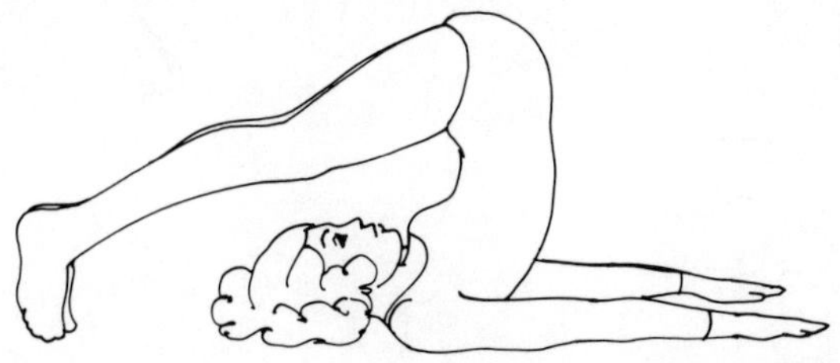

2. *Yoga Full Twist* Sit on the floor with your legs stretched out in front of you. Place the sole of your right foot against the inside of your left thigh. Flex left leg so that you hold your left ankle with both hands. Slowly move your left foot over your right knee and rest it on the floor. Place your left hand on the floor behind you. Move your right arm over your left leg and hold your right knee. Then, slowly twist your trunk and head as far to the left as possible, and hold. Return to forward position and relax. Repeat the same series of movements on the opposite side, breathing slowly and deeply as you move your body, and concentrating on relaxing.

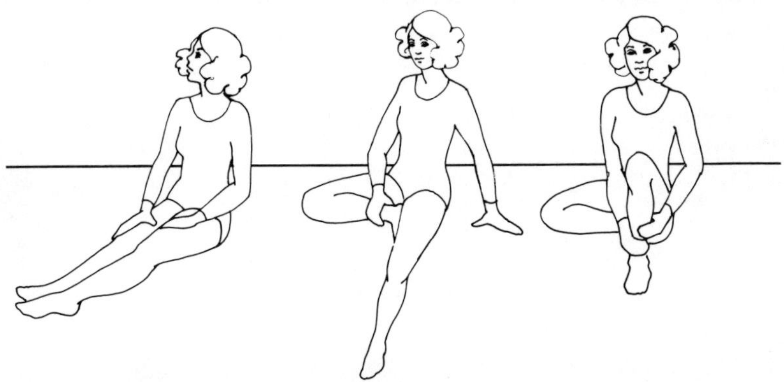

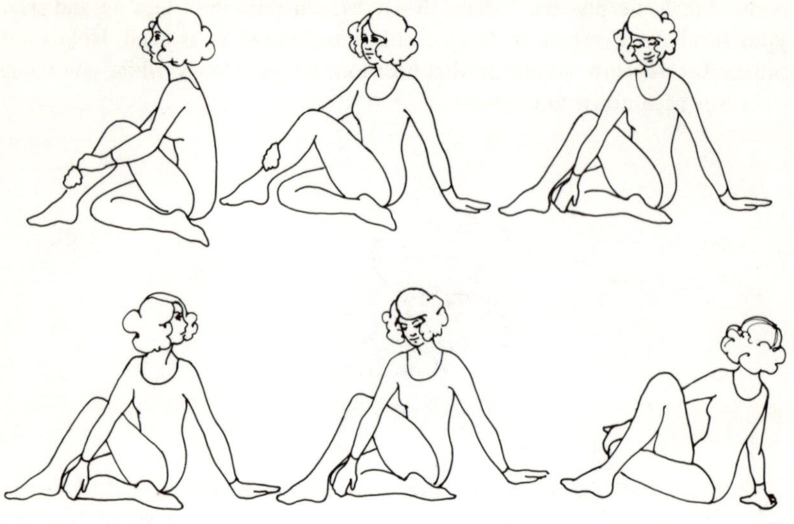

3. *Yoga Neck Roll* From a sitting position, inhale and exhale slowly and deeply as you gradually bend your head forward and touch your chin to your chest. Next gently roll your head to touch your ear to your left shoulder. Then slowly roll your head back, stretching your chin and throat. Slowly roll and twist your head to the right, back, and left positions. With your head in each of the four positions, breathe slowly and deeply. Do this 8 times clockwise, and 8 times counterclockwise.

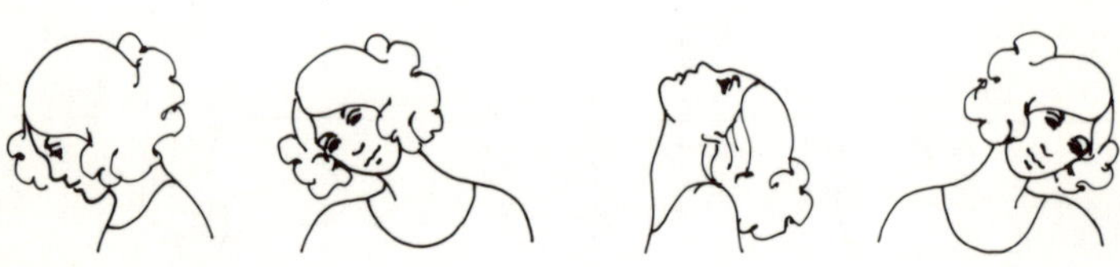

4. *Yoga Seated Chest Expansion*   Sit on the floor cross-legged. Clasp hands behind you and slowly raise your arms. Twist trunk to the left (with arms still raised) and slowly bend forward touching your forehead to your left knee. Slowly straighten up. Twist to the right and touch knee with forehead. Return to an erect position with arms still straight and hands clasped behind you. Breathe slowly and deeply throughout the exercise.

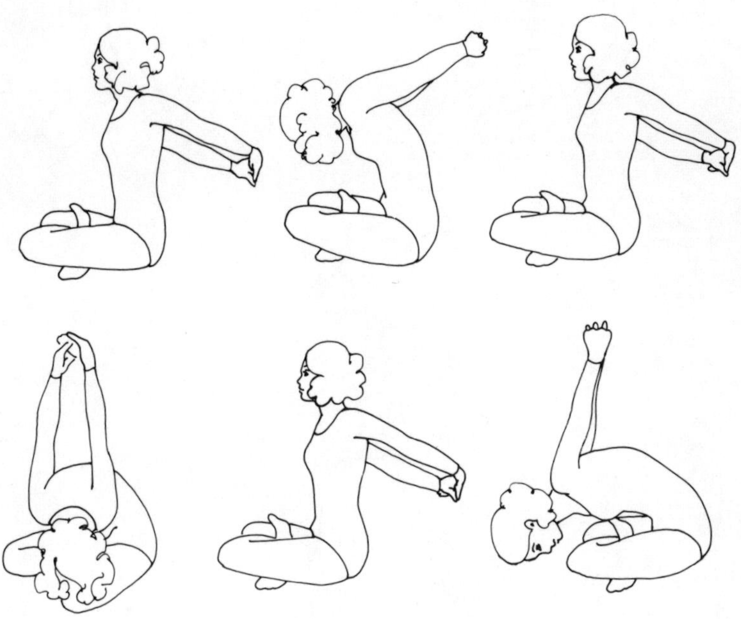

5. *Yoga Full Lotus*   Sitting on the floor place the left foot as high on the right thigh as possible. Place the right foot on the left thigh. Sit erect, breathing slowly and deeply. Making an O shape with the forefinger and thumb of each hand; place them on each folded knee with the remaining three fingers pointed downward. Breathe slowly and deeply throughout each movement, counting slowly to 15 as you inhale, and exhaling for 15

counts. Maintaining the full lotus position, close your eyes and relax as completely as you can. Increase the depth of each breath to 30 counts as you inhale and exhale.

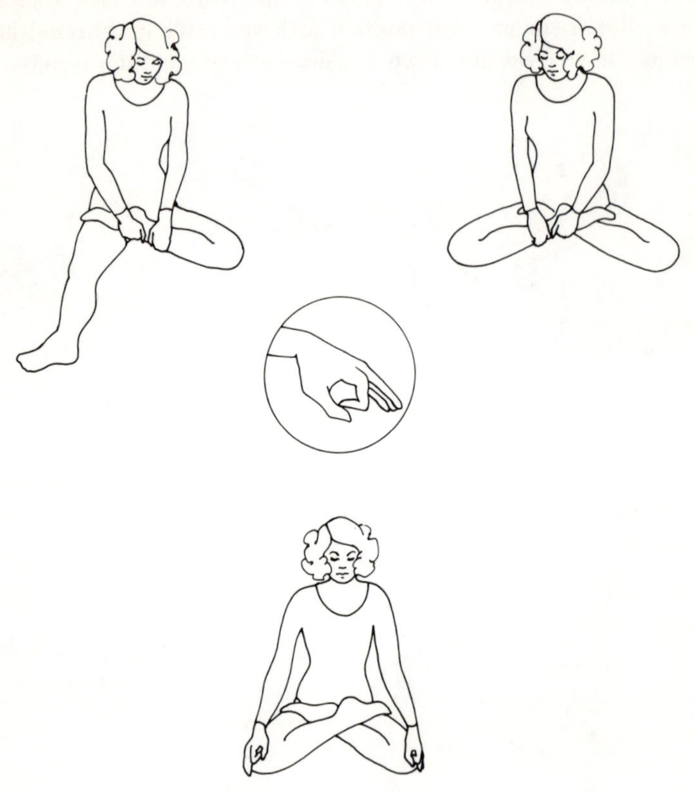

EXERCISES TO RELIEVE MENSTRUAL PAIN

Since menstruation is a normal function of the female body, most women should maintain a normal routine of physical activity during this period. Dysmenorrhea (painful menstruation) can frequently be alleviated by increasing circulation in the lower abdominal region through exercise. In addition, obstetricians believe that exercises that strengthen the abdominal wall facilitate childbirth. Exercises especially designed to strengthen the abdominal wall are found below:

1. *Kitten Arch* Kneel and support your body with your hands. Straighten your back for 4 counts. For another 4 counts, arch your back high and tighten your stomach muscles. Relax. Repeat 15 times.

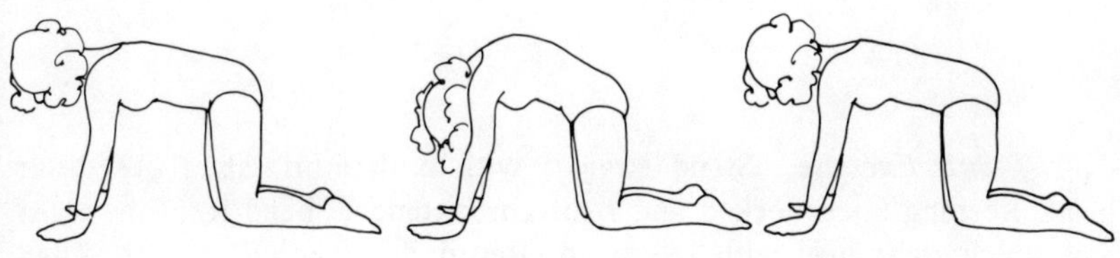

2. *Moser Exercise* Lie on your back with knees flexed and feet flat on the floor. Place your right hand on your abdomen; press and massage your stomach while breathing slowly and deeply.

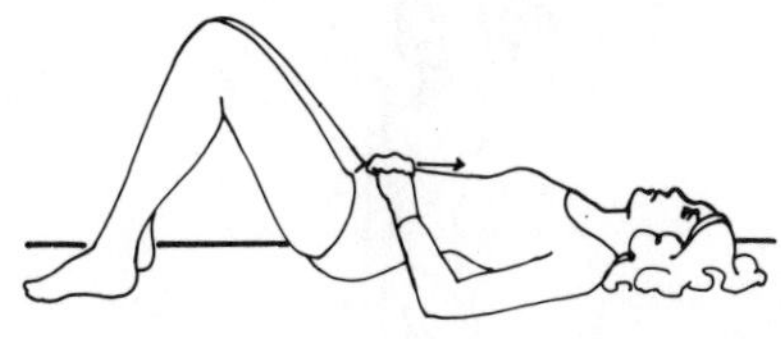

3. *Wall Touch* Lie on your back with arms straight beside body, knees flexed, and your head touching a wall. Bring both knees up over your head to touch the wall; return to place. Repeat 10 times.

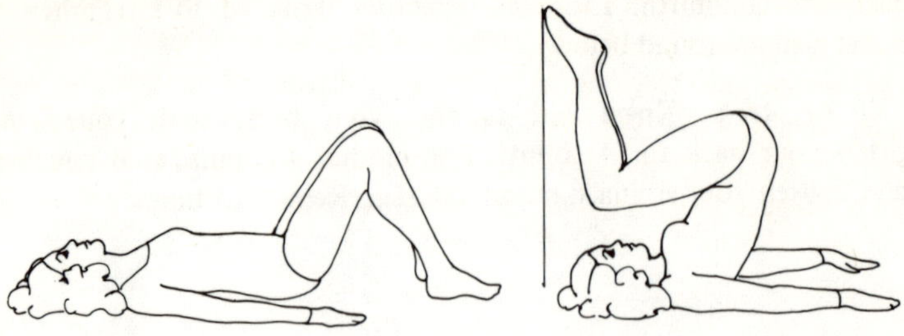

4. *Bolub Exercise*   Stand straight with both arms raised over your head. Keeping knees locked and right arm extended, bend from the waist and touch right heel with left hand. Return to standing position. Then repeat with right hand to left heel, and left arm straight. Relax. Swing both arms forward as you step with your left foot; return to place. Swing both arms forward and step back with your right foot; return to place. Repeat 10 times.

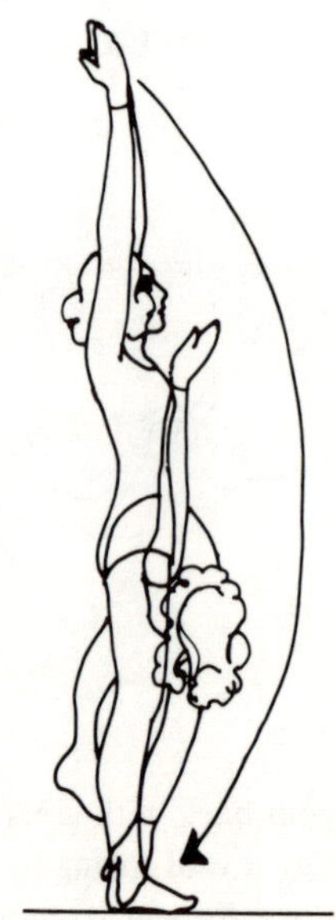

5. *Billig Exercise*   (You should do this exercise at least 10 times daily on each side to receive its greatest benefits.) Stand with your feet together 18 inches from the wall, right hip toward wall. Lock your knees, rotate your hips sideways, and place your right arm horizontally against the wall at shoulder height. Place your left hand against your hip joint. Slowly swing your hip as far forward toward the wall as you can; return to place. Repeat 10 times. Repeat 10 times with left hip toward wall.

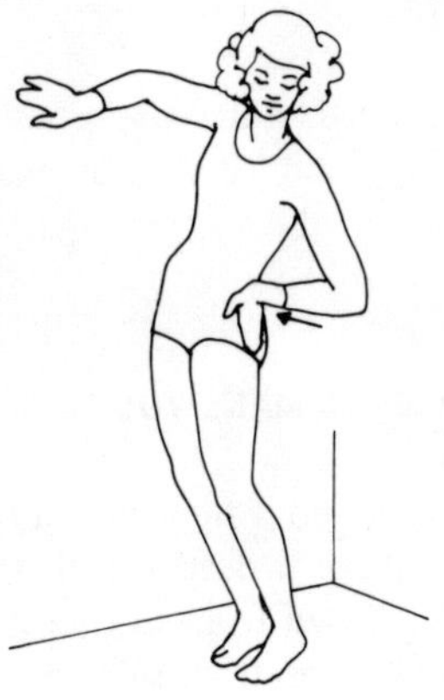

EXERCISES FOR THE NECK, FACE, AND CHIN

1. *Head Tilt*   Sitting in a chair with arms at your sides, drop your head back as far as you can and open your mouth wide. Close your mouth when your head is back the farthest. Repeat opening and closing your mouth 10 times. Raise your head to normal position and relax.

2. *Thinker*   Sit in a relaxed, comfortable position and place your chin in your right palm, right elbow on thigh. With your other hand, forcibly push your head as far to the right as you can, stretching your neck as much as possible. Release your chin and relax. Repeat 5 times with head to each side.

3. *Grinner*   Stretch your face muscles by smiling as widely as you can, then pursing your lips. Repeat 10 times.

4. *Pitty-Pat*   With the back of your hand, tap rapidly under your chin. Relax. Increase speed and intensity to enrich circulation in this area.

5. *Pucker*   To strengthen and firm the area around your chin, press your lips together into a tight pucker. Twist your puckered lips first to the left of your face, then to the right. Repeat 20 times.

6. *Scalper*   Hold your head still; raise your eyebrows and forehead skin. Next, stretch your lips and cheeks far back. Repeat 20 times and increase your speed. Relax.

EXERCISES TO MAKE YOU FEEL GOOD

1. *Pick Me Up*   Stretch on your tip toes and reach toward the sky with your body fully extended. Take a deep breath and tighten your body as much as you can. Then flop down from the waist and bounce three times, letting your body and arms swing from side to side as you exhale slowly. Repeat 10 times.

2. *Flagman*   Stand tall. To the gayest and fastest music you have, alternate flinging your arms up and down as though you had a flag or ribbon in each hand. Move quickly. Next, keeping time to the music, move your imaginary flags in front of you, then fling them out sharply to the sides.

3. *Jumping Jack*   Jump rapidly up and down in place to a fast count or record. Jump rapidly as high as you can, then jump in double time.

4. *Stationary Runner*   Run in place, increasing and decreasing your speed until you are gasping for breath. Time yourself and try to keep going as long as you can. Rest. Increase the time and speed. Do this out of doors often and you will feel exhilarated and refreshed.

5. *Fast Four Moving Parts*   Sit on the edge of a high stool or chair. Move your arms and legs up and down rapidly. This can also be done to music.

HOW TO STAY SLIM AND TRIM FOR LIFE   7

Invest your time and energy in a lifetime physical fitness program. Vow right now to keep active a part of each day for the rest of your life. Youth is a state of mind: you are as old as you feel. Choose the exercise or physical activity best for you and make it a regular part of your life. It might even be fun. People sleep better, think better, digest better, enjoy life more, look, and feel better when they are in good physical condition. Remember, slothfulness is one of the seven deadly sins! You can avoid "hypokinetic disease," the back pains, nervous tension, heart trouble, obesity, and emotional instability resulting from stress — by keeping active.

For refreshment and recreation, take part in sports as well as a vigorous exercise program. Your exercise program will require self-discipline but will increase your enjoyment of active sports and games, and create a more flexible and stronger body. A daily exercise program (at least 15 minutes of vigorous activity), which gives a good workout to all parts of the body is just as important as proper nourishment and proper rest. Learn an individual sport that is completely new and full of pleasure for you. If you sit at a desk all day, choose a sport which exercises your legs: ice skating, roller skating, or bicycling. If you stand most of the day, select gymnastics, swimming, or canoeing, which develop muscular power in your shoulders and trunk. Swimming and jogging are especially good activities; both require strenuous effort and can be done outside — in itself a therapeutic experience.[13] Set your own pace, and above all, have fun.

[13]See the splendid book *Jogging for Fitness and Weight Control,* by Fred Roby and Russell Davis, W. B. Saunders Company, W. Washington Square, Philadelphia, 1970.

The chart below rates (on a scale of 0–100) those activities best for developing endurance, agility, and leg, arm, and abdomen strength. The numbers indicate the relative effectiveness of each sport. Skiing, for example, builds greater endurance than archery; badminton builds more agility than hiking.

Physical Fitness Rating for Individual and Group Sports*

Sport	Endurance	Agility	Legs	Abdomen	Arms
				Strength	
Archery	25	25	25	50	75
Bicycling	50	25	75	25	25
Canoeing	45	45	40	35	35
Hiking	50	25	75	25	25
Horseback riding	25	50	25	50	25
Ice skating	25	75	75	25	25
Mountain climbing	75	75	75	50	75
Roller skating	25	50	75	25	25
Rowing	50	25	50	50	75
Skiing	75	75	75	50	50
Swimming (aquatics)	50	25	50	25	50
Badminton	50	75	75	50	50
Bowling	25	25	50	25	50
Deck tennis	50	75	50	50	50
Golf	25	25	50	25	25
Handball	75	75	75	50	75
Horseshoes	50	25	25	25	50
Paddle ball	50	75	50	50	50
Paddle rackets	50	75	50	50	50
Paddle tennis	50	75	50	50	50
Squash	50	75	50	50	50
Square dancing	50	25	50	25	25
Table tennis	25	50	50	25	25
Tennis	75	75	75	50	50

*Harold Friermood, *The Y.M.C.A. Guide to Adult Fitness* (New York: The Association Press, 1963), pp. 74 and 84.

Select the right sport for you and play it often. Remember that if you go "full throttle" your body will rebel sooner or later, so exercise sensibly. Learn how to make your sleep refreshing and learn how to relax by dividing your time between work and play. Try to avoid worrying, not only for your own sake, but also for those who love you. Worrying is a habit that can be broken. Seek professional help, if necessary.

If you take care of yourself, you'll live a long, happy, and productive life. Be sure to have:

A complete yearly physical examination, preferably by your own doctor who knows your history.

Periodic examinations for physical endurance, strength, and general fitness. (Go to the local Y.W. or Y.M.C.A. or join any night class at your local school or university where a professionally prepared physical educator can help you discover how fit you really are.)

A daily physical exercise program which you do habitually and strenuously enough so that you are gasping for breath and perspiring freely.

Time every day for relaxation and recreative activities which you enjoy.

GLOSSARY 8

Aerobics: With oxygen; doing exercises which cause the lungs to expand more and the heart to pump more blood with fewer strokes.

Calorie: Food units of fuel; a unit of heat needed to raise 1 kilogram (2.2 pounds) of water 1 degree centigrade.

Cholesterol: A fatty substance in the circulatory system which is carried through the blood.

Dysmenorrhea: Painful menstruation.

Ectomorph: Body type (pencil-thin). This type has a frail, underdeveloped body with sloping shoulders, long arms and legs.

Endomorph: Body type (the big square). This type has a square-shape, large frame.

Extension: The straightening of a joint.

Flexibility: Body suppleness.

Flexion: The bending of a joint.

Health: Soundness; freedom from illness.

Isometrics: Pitting one muscle group against its opposite group by moving against it; or resistance against an immovable object.

Isotonics: Equal tension of muscles to produce movement such as calisthenics or weight lifting; exercises which involve free movement.

Joy: Delight; to rejoice.

Leisure: Freedom after school or work. When one is free to do as she wishes.

Mesomorph: Body type (the inverted triangle). This type has a firm, well proportioned body with broader shoulders than hips.

Neuromuscular skill: Learned, coordinated physical movement.

Overload: Working the body harder against resistance or a heavier load by using weights, increased repetitions, or increased speed.

Prone: Horizontal body position with the face down.

Supine: Horizontal body position with the face up.

Visceral: The internal organs in the abdominal cavity.

BIBLIOGRAPHY 9

Books

Barney, Vernon, Cynthia Hirst, and Clayne Jensen, *Conditioning Exercises* (St. Louis: C. V. Mosby, 1965). This book contains excellent photographs and a wide variety of suggested exercises. The chapter on corrective and therapeutic exercise is especially good.

Brean, Herbert, *The Only Diet That Works* (New York: William Morrow Company, 1965). Gives a practical approach to controlling weight through dieting, and suggests ways to remain on the best weight reducing diets.

Cooper, Kenneth and Neirn Brown, *Aerobics* (New York: M. Evans and Company, 1968). This best seller stresses the value of going "all out" as the best way to gain the greatest benefits from exercise programs.

Craig, Marjorie, *Miss Craig's 21 Day Shape-Up Program* (New York: Random House, 1968). A practical approach to body conditioning, attractively written and illustrated.

Davis, Elwood, Gene Logan, and McKinney, *Biophysical Values of Muscular Activity* (Dubuque Iowa: W. C. Brown, 1961). Concerned with the value and results of muscular activity, this is especially good for those seeking scientific information concerning physical activity.

Drury, Blanch, *Posture and Figure Control through Physical Education* (Palo Alto, Calif.: The National Press, 1961). A valuable reference book, especially for movement fundamentals and therapeutic exercise programs.

Good Housekeeping's All Time Best Diets, 200 Great Low-Calorie Recipes Available from Hearst Corporation, 959 8th Ave., New York, N.Y. 10019 (75c per copy). Contains basic facts regarding dieting and nutrition as well as a variety of inexpensive, low-calorie food recipes.

Grossfield, Muriel, *Club 15 Fit for Fun* (Box 1515, Maple Plain, Minn. 55339). A pamphlet especially appealing to teenagers.

Hittleman, Richard, *Be Young with Yoga* (New York: Paperback Library, Inc., 1971). An inexpensive yet valuable book for a beginner in yoga.

Kraus, Hans and Wilhelm Raab, *Hypokinetic Disease* (Springfield, Ill.: Charles C Thomas, 1961). Written by an M.D., this classic book shows the dangers of stress and contains five fitness levels with tests for measuring progress.

Roby, Frederick, and Russell Davis, *Jogging for Fitness and Weight Control* (Philadelphia: W. B. Saunders, 1970). This one is a must for jogging enthusiasts!

Royal Canadian Air Force Exercise Plans for Physical Fitness (New York: Pocket Books, 1962). This book is especially recommended for those seeking a routinized daily exercise program.

Rubin, Theodore, *The Thin Book by a Formerly Fat Psychiatrist* (New York: Trident Press, 1966). An amusing, practical, and valuable "thin" book which suggests ways to capitalize upon human psychological traits to shed "fat" safely.

Shapiro, Sidney, *Swim-nastics* (Hollywood: Creative Sports Equipment, P.O. Box 2244). A program of exercises in the pool designed to increase body flexibility and reduce hard-to-reach areas of the body.

Vannier, Maryhelen, *A Better Figure for You through Easy Exercise and Diet* (New York: Tower Publications, 185 Madison Avenue, 1971). A best seller which illustrates through text and excellent photographs what a daily exercise program can do for one's health, figure, and spirit.

Vannier, Maryhelen and Hally Poindexter, *Individual and Team Sports for Girls and Women*, 2nd Ed. (Philadelphia: W. B. Saunders, 1968). Concise, illustrated instructions for playing a wide variety of sports.

Pamphlets

The following pamphlets are all available free of charge from the National Dairy Council, 111 North Canal Street, Chicago, Illinois.

Calorie-Restricted Diets
Choose Your Calories by the Company They Keep
The Food Way to Weight Reduction
A Girl and Her Figure and You
Go Places, Gal
Guide to Good Eating
Nutrition Handbook for Family Food Counseling
Your Calorie Catalog

Exercise Records for Home and School

"Basic Popular Music," Activity Records, Educational Activities, Inc., Freeport, L. I., New York.

"Chicken Fat," Robert Preston, Capitol Records CF 1000.

"Club 15 Records," Box 1515, Maple Plain, Minn. 55359.

"Feel Good! Look Great!" Debbi Drake, Epic Records, LN 24034.

"Isometrics," Educational Records of America, Inc., Beardsley Station, P.O. Box 6062, Bridgeport, Connecticut.

"Keep Fit," Exercises for Daily Living, Statler Records, N 1009.

"Keep Fit, Be Happy," Bonnie Prudden, Warner Bros. Records, No. B1445 (2 albums).

"Physical Fitness Exercises for Girls," Charles Bucher, Kimbo Records, Box 55, Deal, N.J.

"Reduce in Record Time," Evelyn Loewendahl (with the records comes an illustrated manual), Crown Publishers, New York, N.Y.

"Slimnastics," Charles Bucher, Decca Records. (This is the best of all exercise records, and can be ordered through a local record shop.)

"The Good Housekeeping Plan for Reducing off the Record," Columbia Records No. HL 7143.

"Yoga for Life," Richard Hittleman. Available from Yoga for Health, Box 109, Hollywood, Calif.